To Heidi,

May you always ...
to be your Stronghold.

In His Grip,

Joe

My Stronghold

A Pastor's Battle with Cancer and Doubts

by

Joe Fornear

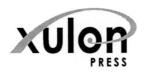

*To the One
who will always have
a strong hold on me.
And to my wife, Terri,
who held me up with human hands.*

Introduction

In December of 2002, I was diagnosed with what doctors believed a terminal case of cancer. Several people who witnessed my free-fall decline and amazing recovery have encouraged me to write. Even if they hadn't, I know the Lord did a unique work, so I feel compelled to tell my story and sing His praises.

I have tried to write the type of book I sought during my bout with cancer. Since I found reading difficult, I preferred smaller chunks, so this book is short with many chapter breaks. Also, though not all cancer patients feel this way, I wanted to know the details of others' struggles. I didn't want to read a sanitized version that left me unprepared for my battle. As a follower of Jesus, I craved a spiritual approach that would give me insight into how He works in the valley of pain. As a student of God's Word, I wanted a balance on the topic of divine healing. Most of the writing on this topic comes from the extremes; either "God guarantees healing" or "God doesn't work that way anymore." As a hurting child of an all-powerful and loving Father, I had to know, did He offer a biblical promise, a guarantee of healing? If He had not made such a guarantee, how did He expect me to get through this trial? I also searched for honesty. Were there others who, like me, did not always handle their cancer very well? On these pages, I may sometimes appear hard on myself or on others. I concluded that if I sugarcoat my story, it will no longer be mine.

Through it all, I discovered more about my weaknesses than my strengths. My takeaway lesson is the theme and the title of this book:

The Lord is strong in spite of my weaknesses. There were times I felt like I had lost my grip. Fortunately, He had a strong hold on me. God is My Stronghold.

Contents

Chapter One

~~~

Friendly Fire

Psalm 139:5-6 - You have enclosed me behind and before, and laid Your hand upon me. Such knowledge is too wonderful for me; It is too high, I cannot attain to it.

During my twelve years of pastoring, I served from time to time at the front lines of the war on cancer. Many heroes of medicine and support have pitched their tents there, but I had never even spent the night. I had done what pastors do. We sit at bedsides. We hold the soldiers' hands. We whisper our prayers, and repeat His comforts. Oh, we care deeply, but before evening falls, most of us retreat quickly to civilian life. During my trips to the front, I considered myself a chaplain, somehow shielded by the rules of engagement. In my subconscious, I wore that special armband with the bright red cross signaling non-combatant status. I was never to be lined up in any crosshairs. Then in late 2002, I received my draft notice. A ticking time bomb had been planted under my arm.

I wish I could say the cancer was a pushover. I've actually developed a kind of spiteful awe of cancer. Its ability to fool the immune system, fly under the radar, and spread rapidly is nothing but diabolical genius. And once some types of cancer gain a foothold, they are very difficult, some would say impossible, for humans to cure. The cancer I had, advanced Stage IV metastatic melanoma falls into this category. Yet things that are impossible with man are possible with

God. Sometimes people tell me they had melanoma too. When I ask for details, they describe a lesion which had been removed from the surface of their skin. Some don't understand the whole staging thing, but before my tour of duty, I didn't either. I would have preferred my education be academic, not experiential. Melanoma attacked fourteen major sites in my body, including stomach, lung, kidney and both the head and tail of my pancreas. Those are some sensitive organs. You might want to hang on to those.

So forgive me if you notice that I suppress a chuckle when someone talks about "beating" cancer. I don't consider myself soft or having a low tolerance for pain, but I really soldiered up with everything I could muster. Still, (permission to speak freely sir) cancer utterly kicked my butt. I was drawn out to the middle of the battlefield, batted around at first, and then dealt some thunderous blows that flattened me. I was like those guys in the war movies, who are shell-shocked into that silent, surreal state. I was able to observe the ongoing battle but felt helpless to respond. Yet as I look back on the run up to my own personal war, maybe the whole thing could have been avoided... but then, I would not have seen such a raw display of divine power.

Now I have revealed my not-so-secret weapon. It's hardly a news flash that a soldier would send up a desperate appeal from his foxhole. "So you prayed a lot? Wow, Joe, good call. How'd ya think of that?" I realize legions of warriors have cried out for healing and not been answered. For some reason, God chose to grant my prayers, well, our prayers. I had a lot of help in that department. So why did God answer our prayers? I will first tell you why not. My story is not "a triumph of the human spirit." It is not "a profile in courage." The headline should not read: "Pastor's Great Faith Lands Divine Healing." I can think of many reasons why others were more qualified to be delivered from death's door. Some had a better attitude. Others had a lot more faith. My five years of seminary training and two decades of teaching on how to be strong in a crisis were evidently not sufficient preparation. My personal weaknesses were rather unflatteringly exposed. Some may think I handled the battle well, but the Lord and I know differently. As you read, you will understand what I mean. If great life crises reveal a person's true colors, then color me gray. My story is not about a courageous escape from the claws of cancer, but a search and rescue operation where the POW is literally carried out of the enemy camp. Why make much of how I handled the cancer? Because I have seen too many cancer patients beat themselves up over their inability to cope. Over time, I learned to embrace this big picture truth: The cancer experience was not about my strong grip on life, but of God's strong hold on me. There was, and still is, a tremendous freedom in resting in that knowledge. Battling cancer is a lot like coping with life in general, neither are do-it-yourself jobs. With the passing of time, it has become clear to me how God intends to use this trial. These days, I have come to regard the cancer as friendly fire from God.

Chapter Two

~~~

Whatever It Is

Job 18:10 - A noose for him is hidden in the ground, And a trap for him on the path.

It all started in September of 2002 when I was 42. I experienced some rubbing under my left armpit and felt a marble-sized lump there. I don't remember the exact day or moment because at the time I wasn't very concerned. You see, about 25 years ago I discovered a pea-sized lump on my chest. I ignored it because it didn't grow. Then during a screening for an insurance policy, I mentioned the lump to an agent who said his underwriter insisted I get it checked out. A doctor declared it a "sebaceous cyst" and said it was harmless. I still have that cyst. It has never grown. About 10 years ago, another lump suddenly appeared on my thigh. I have ignored that lump as well, and it is still there. Hey, so I get little lumps; they're cysts. So when a new lump showed up under my arm, I naturally thought... well, you know. Eventually, I realized this lump was different since it kept growing. So I showed it to Terri, my wonderful and wise wife. I was often reminded throughout the cancer experience, just how wise and wonderful she is. She played a huge role in my story, well, our story. After she felt the lump, she insisted I go to the doctor. So I made an appointment with the kids' doctor since I didn't have a doctor of my own. I rarely needed one.

So in September of 2002, our family doctor felt around my underarm. To him the lump was soft and filled with fluid – like a cyst. Perhaps my history swayed his thinking. I thought the lump was kind of hard, but since it felt as dense as the other benign sebaceous cysts, I wasn't too concerned either. During two separate appointments, my doctor proclaimed confidently, "Whatever it is, it isn't cancer." So he ordered a series of blood tests to search for other causes of swollen lymph nodes, such as infections, mononucleosis, even cat scratch fever. I looked it up; cat scratch is a real disease and not just a Ted Nugent song. He prescribed an antibiotic to knock out any infection. I admit I contributed to the delay in an accurate diagnosis, since I missed a few doses. At a later appointment, three weeks after the first, the doctor recommended I take a stronger, more expensive one-a-day antibiotic. I suppose it was for the dosage-challenged. I determined to get my act together and take the meds consistently. At this point, the lump was continuing to grow, but caused no pain or any other symptoms. The lack of symptoms surely contributed to my laissez-faire attitude. In time, however, my concern grew with the lump. It had grown to the size of a walnut. So my doctor ordered a sonogram to take a closer look.

During the sonogram, in October 2002, the tech did a lot of "hmmming." When I asked what he was seeing, he said with uncharacteristic alarm for a technician, "This is not a cyst, these are lymph nodes!" When I asked about the distinction, he backpedaled quickly. "I am not a radiologist. Let's see what he says. He will give his report to your doctor, and your doctor will contact you in about two or three days." He saved some pictures to disk and shuffled off briskly – a man on a mission. Something significant was discovered, but I would have to wait to find out. Waiting, I would find, is a big part of having cancer. Ultimately there is not a whole lot you can do about the waiting. Fussing didn't help much because, as I would also discover, there are a lot of fussing cancer patients.

After three days of silence about the scan results from my family doctor, I decided to call him. The receptionist seemed fully aware of the report. She put me on hold for a few moments and returned shortly. "Everything is great," she declared. Naturally, I was relieved, but to be sure, I sought further confirmation. "So it is just a cyst, and not lymph nodes?" She said, "That's right." So I said, "OK then, what should I do, make an appointment to have the doctor drain the cyst?" She said, "Yep." She didn't even try to set a time for an appointment, so I figured this was no big medical deal. I just needed to work out a convenient time to get the cyst drained.

Chapter Three

~~~

No Dread

"Such a person will not be overthrown by evil circumstances. God's constant care of him will make a deep impression on all who see it. He does not fear bad news, nor live in dread of what may happen. For he is settled in his mind that God will take care of him." Psalm 112:6-7 (LB)

For most people, convenience is hard to come by, and I was no exception. At the time, I was pastoring Fellowship Bible Church White Rock in Dallas, a church we founded 12 years earlier. I was the regular Sunday preacher and since we were between worship leaders, I led our worship as well. I know, I know, I was doing too much. I wonder if more than any other variable, a compromised immune system from overwork led to my vulnerability to cancer. This cyst thing was just another hassle that I had to fit into my busy and of course, deeply sacred schedule. It is easy to baptize my foibles.

A full month later, my wonderful daughter, Amy, a freshman in high school at the time, contracted a flu bug. The timing of her flu couldn't have come at a better time for me. Accompanying kids to doctor's appointments was not on my normal job description, but I announced I would take her so I could talk to the doctor about the growth of the cyst. It was then about the size of a golf ball.

I remember consoling myself, "It is a good thing the radiologist confirmed this was just a cyst."

After the doctor examined Amy, I piped up. "Hey doc, this cyst has continued to grow. We probably need to go ahead and get it drained." When he felt it, I could tell he was surprised it would continue to expand at such a rate. When I asked about the sonogram results, he left the room. I don't know for certain, but I think that was the first time he read the sonogram report. He returned with a surgeon's phone number and announced it was time to get a biopsy. He added the report concluded the growths were multiple lymph nodes that had swelled. I left his office very concerned and extremely frustrated.

Two more weeks passed before the surgeon had an opening for an initial checkup. He was a young, Type A, straight-shooter who had been voted by his peers as one of the best in Dallas. He reminded me a little of John McEnroe, the tennis player. He flashed this gruff exterior, which after getting to know him, I believe was to prevent him from becoming too attached to patients. When he first saw me he seemed caught up in how husky and strong I appeared. That puzzled me at first, because, well, who cares? Did a football player kick sand on him when he was young? Before the surgery to perform a biopsy, he stressed to the anesthesiologist how big and husky I was. "Make sure you give him enough." I figured my comfort was at issue. On a later date, I mentioned that I revived during an endoscopy (exploratory camera down the throat into the stomach). Then I realized why my size was an issue. He said, "I thought you were going to tell me you clocked the doctor. You know some people revive very violently." All along he had been gauging how much trouble I might be if I awoke during surgery. At my next surgery, my third surgery, he relayed my endoscopy revival story to the anesthesiologist. He never said, "Give him an extra shot; I don't want him coming to and slugging me." Surgeons have a lot to think about. I never imagined defending themselves was one of their concerns.

As he examined me, the theme of my first appointment was the skill level and common sense of my family doctor. "What's his name anyway?" "Cat scratch fever?" "Did anybody ever think to stick a needle in this?" I presumed he meant to pull a quick biopsy. At the time, I was less interested in assessing blame than finding a solution. Yet his reaction told me the size of the mass and the passage of time was a bad combination. Later in February of 2004, after six months of being totally clean of the cancer, Terri and I felt it was crucial for us to have a talk with my family doctor. We asked him to go to lunch and he agreed. We told him what happened with his receptionist. I told him I thought he dropped the ball in my care and that I almost died as a result. He should have immediately called me into the office to review the results of the sonogram, especially since it was such a crucial report. I told him I had decided not to sue him, no matter what his reaction. There is a clear passage in the New Testament about not suing a fellow believer in Christ (1 Corinthians 6:1-8) and he is a believer in Christ and a good guy as well. My motive in confronting him was preventing a repeat with another patient. He was polite but firm, however, insisting his office made no mistakes. He punted on the conversation with the receptionist. Since she wasn't working for him anymore, he couldn't confirm or deny my take on her actions. Afterwards, Terri and I were deeply disappointed, but decided to let it go and move on. Quite unexpectedly, he called us later that evening. He said he had been really pondering my perspective and he began apologizing profusely. He took 100% responsibility for misdiagnosing me and for botching the sonogram report. He said, "I really blew it." His apology released a sense of vindication in me. I was confident that in the future, he would be more conscientious. Some people have asked if he offered me any money. No he didn't; nor did I ask. About a month later, I read in the paper that doctors' insurance companies had identified a proven way to reduce medical malpractice lawsuits. They were encouraging doctors to simply empathize and apologize as much as they could to upset patients. Apparently, people are not as lawsuit-oriented as once thought, they simply want doctors to admit oversights and errors. Human error is part of all of our lives. We just need to learn from those errors. I used to think it would be so stressful to be a doctor, with people's lives depending on your learning curve tacking in the right direction. When you're a plumber, what's the worst that can happen? It's not the end of the world if someone's bathroom rots out because of a leaky pipe you installed. This line of thinking leads me to think about the responsibilities of preaching. As a preacher, you're dealing with more than someone's physical demise, mistakes can have eternal consequences. No wonder preaching is stressful.

By the day of the biopsy three days before Christmas 2002, the lump had become so big I could not touch my elbow to my side without much pain. I decided when I walked around in public, I would hold my other arm out too, in a macho sort of way. The surgeon told me after the surgery that the mass had grown to the size of two baseballs and that he removed the equivalent of one baseball for the biopsy. A pathologist performed some tests while I was still knocked out on the table. The preliminary report was squamous cell carcinoma. When I recovered, the surgeon explained that squamous cell was a type of skin cancer which was very treatable, unlike the most dangerous type - melanoma. So that was good. Still, he said, I should immediately find an oncologist to look into treatment options – perhaps chemo or radiation. He said squamous cell sometimes spreads from the skin down the throat and esophagus or into breathing passages towards the lungs. So I wondered what it was doing under my arm. I remember being grateful that if I had to have skin cancer, at least it wasn't melanoma.

Two days after the surgery, on Christmas Eve morning, I wrote a note to my church. I told them the pathology results and encouraged them to come to the candlelight service that night. I was going to be there, and I just was diagnosed with cancer, so I figured they had no excuse not to show up. Actually, I didn't write that. I was blessed at our church by some of the best people I have ever known. They were a huge support to me and my family. My church family played a pivotal role in my story, well, our story. At the close of the Christmas e-mail, I quoted my son Jesse, who was then a sophomore in high school. "There are a lot of people who get cancer and get through it." Amen, Jesse.

On Christmas Day of 2002, the surgeon called. After further testing, pathologists determined I didn't have squamous cell carcinoma after all, but Stage III metastatic melanoma. He recommended I see an oncologist yesterday. "Metastatic" means on the move or spreading. The cancer cells had spread to my lymph nodes under my arm from another site on my body. They had not been able to locate a "primary" or original source on my skin. I know he felt bad, calling on Christmas, but he was about to go out of town. He agreed to try to help fast track me with tests and oncologists but couldn't promise anything. Some friendly advice for you, as if it were possible to heed: Never get sick on a weekend, and definitely don't ever get sick over the Christmas holidays. The entire medical profession is transported to a distant Christmas planet where they turn off their cell phones and try not to think about desperate patients, jumping up and down on redial buttons.

I found myself clinging to the encouragement in Psalm 112:7, "He does not fear bad news, nor live in dread of what may happen. For he is settled in his mind that God will take care of him" (Living Bible). I need not fear bad news. I need not fear anything. I was in big hands. Good hands.

Chapter Four

~~~

Fellow Patient

Jeremiah 45:3 – "You said, 'Ah, woe is me! For the LORD has added sorrow to my pain; I am weary with my groaning and have found no rest.'"

Here my story takes an ironic and heart-wrenching twist. Just a few months before my diagnosis, my father, Bob, was diagnosed with cancer. Not just any cancer, but of all the possibilities, he had metastatic melanoma. A very small lesion on his back had been pumping melanoma throughout his body. After getting a scan, he was diagnosed Stage IV. The cancer had spread past his lymph nodes to multiple sites, including his lungs, liver and brain. In general, Stage I melanoma is a surface lesion and very treatable. Stage II is a deeper burrowed lesion and is suspect for spreading. A surgeon will usually remove a healthy "margin" of tissue around Stage I or II sites to ensure total removal. I was "only" Stage III. Though the melanoma had passed to my lymph nodes, it seemed to have stopped there and lymph nodes are designed to contain the spread of disease. My dad had an advanced case of Stage IV because of the multiple sites. After some heart to heart discussions with my dad's oncologist, my mother had begun preparing the family for the worst. Then on Christmas Day, I broke an additional load of news to my mom and dad and seven brothers and sisters. "Guess what everybody? I have metastatic melanoma too."

My first reaction was guilt. Irrational, I know, but guilt doesn't always make sense. My dad was in his mid-seventies, and I believed the family should be focused on him. My diagnosis was distracting from what might be his last moments. I experienced additional guilt because I hadn't visited him in Pittsburgh in two years. Terri and I had first moved to Dallas in 1984 so I could attend Dallas Theological Seminary. After I graduated, I started Fellowship Bible Church White Rock in Dallas in 1990. During that time span, I traveled to Pittsburgh at least every other year and sometimes every year. I had already canceled one plane ticket because of my surgeries. Now I had a post-surgery CAT scan scheduled for December 27. The scan was critical to "restage" my case to determine if the cancer had spread. If it had spread, my treatment plan would change considerably, so I needed to stay on track. My concern was whether my dad would still be around if I kept postponing my visit.

I had much more to say than goodbye. I wanted to discuss his soul and the afterlife. As a believer in the Bible, I have some settled beliefs about what happens when we die. I wanted to talk with him about standing before God to give an account for his life, and his relationship with the Savior, Jesus Christ. We had talked before, but not with the certainty I desired. I wanted him to trust only upon the grace and mercy which is offered in Christ. I wanted to know where he stood on these matters. I realize not everyone shares my beliefs. Many people think that everyone who "lives a good life" will go to heaven. From my understanding of the Bible, that is the most unfortunate myth ever perpetuated on the human race. I believe the Bible is clear; there are only two ways to get to heaven. The first way is by living a perfectly sinless life, which means a person has never, ever lied, stolen, cursed, cheated or coveted another's spouse or possessions. The Bible says no one has ever lived such a holy life, except Jesus. I admit I have failed miserably in achieving that first way to heaven. For us sinners there is a clear punishment described in the Bible for our sin. Despite some folk's attempts to discard God's warnings, the punishment is eternal and fiery. Fortunately, there is a "Plan B", a second path to heaven that God has offered. The second way is through the forgiveness God has purchased through the sacrifice of His Son Jesus on the cross. God so loved us that He made a way to forgive us by transferring punishment of our sins onto His Son. So He was punished in our place. But to receive the benefits of this sacrifice, we must each admit our sinfulness and receive Jesus Christ as our personal Savior. No wonder the Bible calls this "good news." It is offered as a free gift. To some, this may seem a simple, even foolish plan, but when one fully considers the sheer holiness of God and the utter sinfulness of man, it makes abundant sense. For more on this, see my tract, The Two Ways To Get To Heaven, which can be found in one of the Appendixes at the end of this book*. I have made sharing this good news part of my life's purpose. I feel it is not only a privilege but an obligation to share these message with others. So how could I neglect to make the trip to clarify these truths with my own father? Talking over the phone had become difficult. There were too many visitors and hovering nurses. But I decided to trust the Lord with my dad's soul and his salvation, knowing He could send hundreds of people to make sure my dad was properly prepared to meet Him. Looking back, it would have been foolish to make the trip in my condition. My sister put it well, "We don't need both of you to die – stay down there and get better."

A reluctant respect for melanoma began to settle in. I was glad my family didn't shield me from the realities of my dad's decline. I was not blind-sided by the intensity of the disease. I tried to research all I could. The studying didn't last long because the internet is not exactly a fountain of hope for later stage melanoma patients. The five year survival rate for advanced Stage IV is roughly 3 to 6%. There are, however, many medical and news articles on promising clinical trials. As I eagerly dove into these hopeful claims, I would discover the "amazing progress" was often an addition of three or four months to the life of a patient. Not exactly the progress I had in mind. I imagine some doctors regret the rise of the internet. Patients gain just enough knowledge to second guess their advice. By this point in my struggle, the hope this would be a quick or easy battle had disappeared. As the stories of my dad's condition grew worse, I couldn't help wonder where melanoma was dragging me.

*The tract, "The Two Ways To Get To Heaven," can also be found on Stronghold Ministry's website at: www.mystronghold.org/Docs/ The_Two_Ways_To_Get_to_Heaven.pdf.

Chapter Five

~~~

Questions

Job 7:20 - "Have I sinned? What have I done to You, O watcher of men? Why have You set me as Your target, So that I am a burden to myself?"

There are 1 million new cases of skin cancer every year. A huge percentage of those diagnosed have opportunity to catch the disease in Stage I or II. I found myself wondering why the cancer skipped the early stages and advanced directly to my lymph nodes, which is Stage III. I had thought melanoma always formed a surface lesion on the skin, but learned it is "not uncommon" to have an original source, or "primary" on the skin. In these cases, some oncologists believe the immune system manages to fight the melanoma off the surface of the skin, but fails to prevent the spreading of cells to the rest of the body. This stealth effect is particularly dangerous since early detection is one of the greatest tools in fighting melanoma. In these types of cases, diagnosis and treatment are most always delayed. Cancer can really "fly under the radar." I have yet to see published skin cancer advice which warns of the possibility of the disease going straight to your lymph nodes. I have a layman's primer at the back of this book in one of the appendixes. Nor have I ever read that we should beware that potentially deadly lesions can disappear as quickly as they had formed. I have met two melanoma patients whose primary lesion was on, or in, their eyeball. There are also cases of women having primary lesions on skin that is covered by their bathing suit. This leads some doctors to conclude ultraviolet rays can penetrate clothing. We recently heard of a woman who found a lesion on her private part. Also some people have been diagnosed on the soles of their feet, others on the palms of their hands, even some on their finger or toenail beds. I know of two babies who were born with melanoma. Also, until my dad's story I always thought a dangerous lesion had to be large. So I mention these rarer cases to help spread the word. Much more vigilance in caring for our skin is required today. Nationally, there are more new cases of skin cancer each year than the combined incidences of breast, prostate, lung and colon cancers.

I had another more penetrating personal question; had I brought this disease on myself? In many ways I was a prime candidate for melanoma. Every dermatologist or oncologist I have ever seen requires patients to complete a lengthy survey (often 30 or 40 pages) on their lifetime relationship with the sun. The initial questions deal with family history, since melanoma seems to have some hereditary aspects. My extended family picked up on this without requiring any statistical proof. After my dad and I were both diagnosed within months of each other, business got very brisk at Pittsburgh area dermatology offices. The genetic connection was brought home even more dramatically when I met a young child who was born with a lesion on the back of her hand. Her grandfather had a lesion in almost exactly the same location! The skin cancer surveys also ask, "Are you fair skinned?" and "Do you burn easily?" Pffft. I can't even begin to count the number of sunburns this light skinned, blue-eyed boy has had. Sunburn was a rite of summer passage in my younger days. If you weren't red, you might as well be dead. You clearly weren't enjoying your summer. I especially remember achieving that familiar cherry hue after playing in the lake or fishing all day at Conneaut Lake Park, my family's annual vacation destination. Actually, I was outdoors all summer long for most of my life. I played baseball since I was six years old through college, and even for a few years after college in summer leagues. There were also a couple of summers of vanity in high school when I would lay out in the sun after drenching with baby oil. I thought the chicks dug it.

(My wife said I could write that). I worked outdoor construction jobs every summer beginning freshman year in high school and all the way through college. Upon high school graduation, I moved south to live in Florida for five months. Working as a rough frame carpenter for eight to ten hours, I would finish most days throwing Frisbee on Daytona Beach. I made my living after college and during seminary years working construction. During my bi-vocational first two years of the church, I regularly spent long days working under the Texas sun. I replaced more than a few Texas roofs as a contractor, sometimes reroofing houses by myself. I reroofed my own homes three times. To top off this sun overdose, my favorite hobby was fishing. I have been told, by some fairly avid fishermen, that it is not easy fishing with me, because I stay out too long. My fishing theory is that fish have to eat, so if you wait them out, eventually they will bite. In my adult years, I grew diligent in using sunscreen while fishing, but I admit, I wouldn't reapply every few hours. So genetics, occupation and lifestyle combined to form the perfect storm for melanoma and me.

I certainly can't blame my parents since knowledge about skin cancer had not sufficiently evolved during my childhood. Perhaps I could have sidestepped the cancer if during my adult years, I had not minimized warnings. I am comfortable taking 100% of the blame for not taking better care of my skin. At first it bugged me to think families were probably sitting around their dinner tables discussing my situation. I imagined parents saying, "Mr. Joe was out in the sun way too much and see; this is what happens. So you listen to us the next time we tell you to use sunscreen." We have a strong inclination to determine the exact cause of others' sufferings. If we can pinpoint the cause, we feel empowered to avoid the consequences. There is some truth there. There is also value in being a negative example, so yes, please use a lot of sun screen and don't stay out in the sun too long, like me.

I also believe what God allows, He also determines. He could have easily circumvented my irresponsibility. He could have allowed the cancer to stay on the surface of my skin to give me time to treat it. I once read the human body fights off a cancer attack 30,000 times in one's lifetime. So the Lord through the immune system He designed is constantly preventing people's cancer. He could have allowed my body to fight it off just one more time. Well actually, He did. I mean much sooner. I wonder about this too: why have some serial sunbathers continually managed to dodge the melanoma bullet? Some have fairer skin than I, more vulnerable genetics, and also were far less responsible with sunscreen. The fact is we are always dodging bullets from dumb decisions. Driving too fast for conditions; running red lights; eating poorly; living recklessly; we are all on borrowed time. When I think about it, God was extremely gracious to allow me to survive my teen years.

I don't believe I was being punished though. I have spoken to more than one cancer patient who was not so sure. Technically, I deserve a far worse, everlasting suffering because of the multitude of my sins. God would be totally justified in instantly sending me straight to hell, but I believe He washed my sin away through Jesus' death on the cross. In my struggles with the "why" question, His mercy was never an issue, only His purposes. I am convinced He had higher purposes in allowing the cancer. All of those purposes will be revealed in eternity, but some of the reasons have become obvious.

Chapter Six

~~~

Invader

Exodus 15:9 - The enemy said, "I will pursue, I will over-take, I will divide the spoil; My desire shall be gratified against them; I will draw out my sword, my hand will destroy them."

The cancer had managed a surprise attack, my Pearl Harbor, but finally a counterattack was planned. Right after my first surgery in December 2002, my surgeon recommended an oncologist. He was a kind and sharp man of Indian descent, but his accent was thick and I often had trouble understanding him. I had so many questions too, and I wanted to talk a lot. Though he made some decent efforts, I often felt under informed. Frankly, he seemed overextended to me. He had two offices in two different locations which were about an hour's drive apart. He would return my calls on his cell phone while driving between offices, which made him even harder to understand. I think he drove a convertible too. The accent was not the only barrier that made communication difficult. This experience was so unexpected and upsetting to me. Being an oncologist would be tough. Most of their patients perceive themselves to be on the precipice of life and death because, well, they are. The deluge of questions has to be draining, especially because no one really wants to hear some of the answers. He was confident, however, in advising my next step. I should have a second surgery to remove the remainder of the lymph nodes under my arm and then follow up with an immune system drug called Interferon. This, he said, was "the standard of care" for Stage III melanoma patients. Interferons are natural proteins produced by our immune systems to knock out viruses, parasites and tumor cells. They prevent viruses and tumors from reproducing because they activate the body's protective T cells. I was relieved that my doctor's top recommendation was a natural treatment, since I was concerned about long term side effects of harsh cancer drugs. Yet in the end, I never received any Interferon treatments.

After the first surgery, I had a PET scan and an MRI to rule out brain metastasis and to restage me. PET is an acronym for "positive emission tomography." A radioisotope is mixed with glucose and injected into the bloodstream. Our bodies convert all food into glucose to feed our cells. Since fast growing cancer cells drink up glucose at a higher rate, the radioisotope becomes more concentrated in cancer cells. The scanner detects higher radiation levels from clusters of cancer cells and pinpoints their location(s). The PET scan lasts about 35 minutes. When you have melanoma, they also scan your legs and feet, which is another 25 minutes. I began to learn the meaning of the old saying, "The cure is worse than the disease." During a PET, the arms must be placed above the head. The position was a problem for me since it ripped apart the sutures and scar tissue under my arm.

The mass continued to blow up under my arm. There was a constant tingling sensation in the area. I realized it was due to blood gushing through rapidly multiplying cancer cells. The mass was bulging out both sides of my underarm. In the front, it had grown up onto my upper chest and shoulder, reaching all the way to my collar bone. During an office visit two weeks from the date of the first surgery, the surgeon was shocked by the size of the mass. He figured it could only be due to a build up of lymphatic fluid caused by removing so many lymph nodes. So he repeatedly tried to drain the area with a syringe, but found only rock solid tumor everywhere he pierced. Yes, tumors have nerve endings. By the time he resected, or removed the mass in surgery, it had grown to 8" x 6" x 4" - roughly the size of a banana bread pan. He said the tumor had grown so fast the mass was "necrotic" or dead on the inside. The outer layer of cells had been greedily siphoning all of the blood supply and the inner cells had died for lack of blood. He could not get over the aggressiveness of my case. He warned me to get the strongest systemic chemo I could find, immediately. But before he could hand me off, he would be pressed into service one more time.

After the second surgery and before beginning chemical treatment, I was required to have another PET for restaging. It revealed a quarter-sized lesion inside my stomach. Since the cancer had spread past my lymph nodes, so I was now classified as Stage IV. At least, everyone said, there was only one place the cancer had spread. The doctors recommended an endoscopy in which a camera is inserted into the throat and down into the stomach. A biopsy of the lesion could be removed and studied. I awoke during the procedure to a doctor holding a contraption that looked like a bicycle handle bar with a remote control joystick mounted on it. I didn't think I was supposed to be awake, so I tried to make some small talk with the doctor to let him know I was awake. He wasn't looking at my eyes because he was staring down at a video monitor on the side of my bed. So I said, "Do people wake up during endoscopies very often?" When I spoke, he jumped back in fright and was caught totally off guard. He recovered nicely though and said, "Oh well, we are done anyway." I don't think that was entirely true. I'm just glad he didn't have someone bonk me with a big rubber mallet to put me out again; "He woke up. Give him another whack!" Another surgery was scheduled to have the affected part of my stomach removed. The surgeon estimated he would remove one-third of my stomach. I could tell he thought we were only buying some time. I told myself, sometimes God takes His time.

Chapter Seven

~~~

Under the Knife

Luke 2:35 - And a sword will pierce even your own soul.

To this point I had been fitting treatment into my schedule. I was keeping up with church duties fairly well. I was determined not to let the cancer impact my kids too adversely. There were signs my son, Jesse, was growing more concerned. On several occasions, when Terri and I would sit the kids down to give them an update, I could see him brace himself against his chair. He told me later he struggled with the relevancy of routine matters like sports and school against a backdrop of life and death. His grades suffered, but he seemed more inspired in his basketball games. He was definitely more aggressive and his coach played him more. He also found an outlet in his computer gaming. He got really good at a game ironically called, Counterstrike. My daughter, Amy, was always confident I would be fine. She has been the family optimist and has a simple trust in the Lord. I was hoping the developments in my life wouldn't overwhelm her tender faith. I made a goal to attend every high school basketball game the kids played. Jesse was on the boy's JV team and Amy was on the girl's freshmen team. I remember running through parking lots to gyms on cold, wet evenings, pulling my shirt away from the incision under my arm, to prevent rubbing and sticking. At this point though, I could no longer fit cancer treatment into life. It had become a full time job. I thought of the airline's advice, "Put your own oxygen mask on before you try to help your children." I was not happy about the shift of focus though. My life had begun to spin out of control, at least my control, and a battle of the wills had begun. I played the fussy toddler and God the patient Father.

The first opening to schedule the stomach surgery was a Monday morning, the day after the Super Bowl in 2003. I noticed the timing conflict too late. We had scheduled a big Super Bowl party at the church. I should have allowed one more day because preparation on the night before the surgery required drinking a fluid that empties the stomach. So I had to leave the big party after the first half. As I sat in the bathroom "preparing," I had the sense that my life was about to become very complicated. Everything was progressing at warp speed. I still had a drain attached under my arm from the second surgery and couldn't remember any instructions about removal. It was a plastic suction pump which was shaped like a hand grenade. It connected to a quarter inch plastic tube that was buried in my incision area. I was to squeeze the bulb now and then to drain lymphatic fluid since its route had been interrupted by the removal of lymph nodes. I decided to yank out the tube since it hadn't been draining well anyway. As I slowly pulled it out, I was surprised that it was about 18" longer than I thought. It had been curled up in a tight coil under my skin. The drain must have been clogged because when the end of the tubing cleared the incision, fluid shot out from it with enough force to spray the bathroom mirror. The flow receded to a drip in a few seconds. I was hoping I had done the right thing, but I thought, "What are they going to do to me?"

The next morning, the surgeon removed some parts, including a third of my stomach, a fist-sized lymph node in my abdomen, and a section of my omentum. The omentum is an internal fat layer located on the inside of the abdominal wall which cushions and insulates internal organs. When I revived, I was told pathologists still weren't certain I had melanoma. All of the biopsy reports still concluded "weak for melanoma." They were perplexed by the lack of clarity and wondered if I might have stromal stomach cancer instead. My oncologist said, "This might be some really good news – if you have to have cancer, you want to have stromal stomach cancer." A new wonder drug, called Gleevec, knocks out stromal with minimal side effects. The hospital sent off a biopsy to a highly regarded pathology specialist in stomach cancer. We prayed diligently and crossed our fingers and toes that I had stromal. It took almost two weeks for a response but the specialist came back with the same conclusion, "weak for melanoma." This news totally deflated my remaining human optimism. Terri's confidence had taken a big hit too while she was waiting for me to come out of the surgery. Usually she had several friends from church sitting with her in the waiting room. For some reason she was alone for a time on the day of my stomach surgery. She tells what happened:

"There was an older man and his daughter waiting for his wife to come out of surgery. It was so quiet; I couldn't help hearing their discussion. The husband said, 'I dread this disease, every time they go in to take some out, it just seems to spread more and more.' I was wondering which disease. His next words were, 'Melanoma has no end.' This man had no idea my husband was under the knife right then for the same disease. Anxiety swelled up in my heart. I played out the next ten years in my mind. I would be totally alone. I was not ready for this battle in this waiting room. I had not put on the shield of faith. The lion had been waiting for me there, roaring loud and clear that I was not going to make it. Joe's stomach was being cut. I was being cut in my heart. Nobody saw it happening. No doctor was going to talk to those waiting for a report on this bloodless surgery. This battle was only seen in the invisible world, where dark spirits battle over beliefs in God. Is He good no matter what? Does he provide and care for me in my unseen future? Will He carry me through the next hour?"

Terri's account reminds me of the angel Gabriel's comments to Mary, that her heart would be pierced along with Jesus' heart. His heart was literally pierced, hers figuratively. In those days I often looked at Terri and realized if I were to pass away, she would be left "holding the bag." I could feel the storm gathering force in the distance, but how do you hold back a storm? I was trying.

Chapter Eight

~~~

The Support

Exodus 17:11-12 - So it came about when Moses held his hand up, that Israel prevailed, and when he let his hand down, Amalek prevailed. But Moses' hands were heavy. Then they took a stone and put it under him, and he sat on it; and Aaron and Hur supported his hands, one on one side and one on the other. Thus his hands were steady until the sun set.

My recovery from the stomach surgery began well. The incision and my insides were sore as expected, so I liberally used the "patient-controlled" morphine drip. The drip machine is designed to measure and limit intake, but also to allow a patient to skip doses if their pain is not bad. There is a timer which beeps when the machine will allow another dose, but I was not skipping any doses. As soon as I heard the beep, I would instantly push the button for as much relief as possible. Then, two days after the surgery, a nurse told me she had seen little old ladies use half of the morphine I was using. It felt like she was questioning my manhood. I suppose she was questioning my womanhood too, if I was weaker than little old ladies. I quickly locked and loaded the old ego. I was going to cut out the self-pity routine and the morphine. "Just give me a towel to bite on." So for a day I writhed on the bed, trying to match the toughness of the little old ladies on my floor. The next day I was assigned to a nurse who was one of those really good, experienced and efficient types, who want you to know that they are really good, experienced and efficient. A side note to all of you good, experienced and efficient types: we notice, you can relax. Anyway, I am confident the Lord sent her to me. She hit the roof when she heard what the other nurse had said. So the happy flow of morphine resumed.

There were some definite highlights of my stay at Doctor's Hospital. I felt so supported by friends, family and church. One huge blessing was a visit by some of my basketball buddies. I had been playing pick up basketball with them for several years and I know how much they look forward to playing. Instead of playing one day, several of them agreed to visit me. They always put me in good spirits, usually through making fun of each another. One said with a straight face while rubbing his nose in that suggestive, helpful kind of way, "Hey, you got something in your nose." He was referring to the half inch nose tube which was siphoning surgery fluid from my stomach into a bag. Another group of men came to visit me, the Ironmen. These were my son's high school friends with whom I had been meeting weekly for a Bible study for the last four years from 7th grade. We didn't meet during that year, their junior year while I was battling cancer, but we picked up again in their senior year. I was blessed they were looking after a wounded soldier. I should not have been surprised, because they were great guys and their parents are kind and sensitive people. Still their visit caught me off guard and I was very emotional after they left. They wanted to help in a practical way. I immediately thought of the exterior of our house which badly needed painting. They offered to do it, and initially I was inclined to agree. Then I had second thoughts when I imagined how the house and yard would look after a paint battle. So they raised a bunch of money so I could hire a painter.

Often great blessings came from unexpected sources. One woman, whom I barely knew from our kids' grade school, sent me a weekly encouragement card. She was a busy mother and a doctor's wife, so she had a thousand greeting card options. So her thoughtfulness seemed a God thing to me. He had put it on her heart to care in such a faithful way. More unexpected kindness came from an old friend and high school basketball buddy with whom I had minimal contact since high school. He wrote me 30 different e-mails to cheer me up. He would write about our high school exploits, "Remember when..." He also sent encouraging quotes from Oswald Chamber's classic daily devotional, "My Utmost For His Highest." The best part of our reconnection was our focus on spiritual issues with the Lord. In high school, we didn't spend much time talking about Jesus. Once I tried to convince him the most reasonable explanation for Jesus' superior powers was that He came from an advanced civilization in outer space.

There were many other surprise blessings, but one of the most noteworthy came in early June of 2003, during one of my lowest points. I was bald and emaciated and sitting in a wheelchair in a crowded hospital waiting room. A 6 years old boy grew more and more taken by my appearance. He crawled up on a chair facing me and stared at me for several seconds. He climbed down a few times to trade whispers with an adult who sat across the room. Then he would return and resume the staring. It was awkward at first, but eventually I was equally fascinated with him. I tried to guess what in the world he was thinking. Then I sensed his emotion morphing from what seemed like pity to admiration. Finally, he spoke, "Mister, I'm sorry you are so sick. I hope you get better." It was a small thing to say, but "out of the mouth of a babe," it was a huge comfort. It was as if the Lord was telling me to hang in there, He knew it was hard.

On the third day in the hospital after my stomach surgery, I could not get warm, so I had the room temperature increased. I began to sweat profusely, so I had the thermostat turned backed down. They took my vitals and said I had an infection. A blood sample revealed it was a staph infection, but fortunately it was the low severity type. They said I probably brought the staph infection into the hospital since there was a high culture reading found in the incision under my arm. They gave me some antibiotics, but before they kicked in, the high fever and morphine combined to produce a series of bizarre and surreal nightmares. I dreamed of lightning fast, technicolor demons that pursued me through the streets of some city. The figures would morph and dematerialize, flashing to new locations to strike blows at me as I ran. I was like Kung Fu fighting and I was getting in some good kicks myself. I knew the dream was symbolic of what I was feeling, but when I fully awoke, all I could say was, "Wow." As in, bad trip. I decided to cut way back on the morphine. As a bonus, I'm sure I improved my reputation with a nurse and some little old ladies on the 6th floor. The next morning at dawn, they quarantined me and my room. A cleaning lady scrubbed down every inch of my room with a disinfectant. Soon the fever broke and I felt much better. I was very glad because I wanted to concentrate on getting out of the hospital, to jump on a plane to Pittsburgh to see my dad.

Chapter Nine

~~~

Cursing the Distance

Job 3:1-4 - Afterward Job opened his mouth and cursed the day of his birth. And Job said, "Let the day perish on which I was to be born, And the night which said, "A boy is conceived." May that day be darkness; Let not God above care for it, Nor light shine on it.

Early in February 2003 on my fifth day in the hospital in Dallas, my mother called me from the hospital in Pittsburgh where my dad was being treated. All seven brothers and sisters and spouses were gathered there with my dad. She began unfolding the scenario I did not want to hear. My dad was in critical condition. His melanoma had spread so rapidly that his systems were beginning to shut down. He was in a lot of pain, but with his age and his blood pressure, giving him enough morphine to lessen his pain might shut him down completely. She stressed the doctors wanted to keep him comfortable, and I of course agreed. I was surprised, however, that my dad was able to talk much on the phone. Not only was he talking clearly, he was amazingly upbeat. It was probably the morphine talking. He told me he had an appointment that Monday to start a promising new melanoma trial with Dr. John Kirkwood, a renowned melanoma researcher out of The University of Pittsburgh Cancer Institute. He was confident he was going to make it. As I hung up, I was confused at the disparate pictures my parents had painted. Still I knew without divine intervention, my father's passing would be very soon. So I fervently asked the Lord to grant a delay so I could make the trip.

The next morning, I was pondering how to convince my doctor to release me and clear me for immediate travel. I heard a tremendous boom outside. It really startled me, but I thought a truck had dropped a dumpster in the parking lot. Later a nurse told me the noise was from the explosion of the space shuttle. It was heard all over northeast Texas. I clicked on the TV to watch the coverage and like many Americans, I was deeply grieved over the tragedy. I wondered where Terri was, since she had always arrived at the hospital much earlier in the mornings. I figured she was delayed by the shuttle news coverage. But when she walked into the room I could see on her face that the grief was much more personal. My dad had passed in the night.

Everyone knows their dad will die, but I had just had an upbeat conversation with him 12 hours ago! How could he have declined so fast? This was my dad, tougher than life, the Steel City man. One day he kicked a football way over the top of the telephone poles. More than once he broke bricks for us out in the backyard. He drove himself to the hospital after an electric power drill tore off his finger. Surely he could have fought a few more days until I got there. Surely God could have helped him.

When the surgeon arrived to check on me, he was extremely compassionate after hearing about my dad. He agreed to release me early, but he advised me not to travel. The funeral was in just four days, and deep down I knew I was not ready to fly. I had just begun to get out of bed on my own. The doctor said if I absolutely insisted on going, he would give me an emergency hotline number to reach him. After talking with the family, I decided not to go. I still think that was the right decision. I would need all my strength for my own battle.

Still, if the Lord had delayed my father's death just two or three more days, I could have gone to the funeral. So why didn't He? I turned to the book of Job, who experienced the perfect storm of trials. He endured a loss of all his possessions, and the death of all ten of his beloved children. On top of that he was given a horrible skin disease. Then his best friends blamed him for all of his troubles, in a loving, concerned kind of way. They were tried to get him to admit some deep dark sin that was surely the root cause of his suffering. The story of Job reminds me of a song from an old Arlo Guthrie album called Alice's Restaurant. In one song, Arlo muses about "the last guy":

> During these hard days and hard weeks, everybody always has it bad once in a while. You know, you have a bad time of it, and you always have a friend who says. "Hey man, you ain't got it that bad. Look at that guy." And you look at that guy, and he's got it worse than you. And it makes you feel better that there's somebody that's got it worse than you. But think of the last guy. For one minute, think of the last guy. Nobody's got it worse than that guy. Nobody in the whole world. That guy...he's so alone in the world that he doesn't even have a street to lay in for a truck to run him over.

I think Job's story is included in the Bible so that he will forever be "the last guy." No matter what we are going through, the pain of our circumstances cannot begin to approach the torture that went on in that righteous man's soul. Granted, it's a strange comfort, to be consoled by another's misfortune, but Job's story nullifies one of our greatest obstacles - self-pity. There is someone out there who has gone through far more troubles than I ever will, and he handled it with grace and dignity. So if things go deep south on you, try consoling yourself with Job's good attitude towards his trials. It worked for me. Despite his unimaginable pain, Job never spoke evil of God. His wife even encouraged him to curse God as a sure way to end his nightmare. She said, "Why do you hold fast to your integrity? Why don't you just curse God and die?" Job didn't though. He did, however, curse something. Before my ordeal, I had never really focused on this aspect of his response. Job cursed the day of his birth, lamenting that he had ever been born. As I read and reread his outcry, I felt an overwhelming urge to curse something. Honestly, I wasn't mad at God or the doctors or myself; I was mad at the circumstance of my inability to travel. So for a few days, I found solace in cursing the distance between me and my family in Pittsburgh. Somehow, it helped. Don't ask me to explain.

I heard reports about my dad's funeral from family members and I watched a video of the service. Of course it wasn't the same. Even so, I never got to say goodbye in person. As I mentioned previously, my evangelist side was in overdrive about my father. I had been concerned about his soul, as I would be for anyone, but especially someone I loved. Within the week I heard some really good news on this front. My aunt told me she spoke to my dad before he died to ask if he had invited Jesus Christ into his heart as his Savior. My dad replied, yes, he had. So I was tremendously relieved that he had indeed received the free gift of salvation before he passed over. It was a huge relief to know God hadn't "needed" me after all. I will soon be reunited with my dad in heaven. When I see him, I doubt we'll trade melanoma war stories. Those days will be forgotten. We will be forever encompassed and caught up in the perfect presence of God.

Though it's now over six years since he died, whenever I think very long about missing his funeral and not saying goodbye, I'm still overcome with emotion. I don't know exactly why. I know it's some sort of closure thing. I have no doubt many others feel this way about loved ones. I never had someone that close to me pass away with such frustrating timing. Maybe it's supposed to feel this way.

Chapter Ten

~~~

Im-patient

Job 4:1-6 - Then Eliphaz the Temanite answered, "If one ventures a word with you, will you become impatient? But who can refrain from speaking? Behold you have admonished many, And you have strengthened weak hands. Your words have helped the tottering to stand, And you have strengthened feeble knees. But now it has come to you, and you are impatient; It touches you, and you are dismayed. Is not your fear of God your confidence, And the integrity of your ways your hope?"

Eleven days after the stomach surgery, on Valentine's Day, I went again to see my oncologist. I thought he was going to begin Interferon treatments. Instead, he told me Interferon is usually given to second stage patients who have deep lesions removed and to third stage patients who have lymph nodes removed. It is an "adjuvant" drug, designed to prevent relapse and given after surgical removal of melanoma. But because of the aggressiveness of my Stage IV cancer, he felt I needed something systemically stronger than Interferon because they couldn't keep cutting on me. He said metastatic melanoma is very resistant to conventional chemotherapies and radiation. So he suggested a potent drug called high dose Interleukin-2 (IL-2), which supercharges the immune system to fight off the cancer. The five year survival rate after receiving this drug is 6% which is not very good, but he said it was "the standard of care" for my situation. He said the side effects of the drug are pretty rough but I was young and strong. During early clinical testing of high dose IL-2, several people died from renal (kidney) failure, so close monitoring in the hospital during treatment is mandated by the FDA. More than five years later, my oncologist told me that high dose Interleukin-2 is no longer the main treatment option for Stage IV metastatic melanoma. Low dose IL-2 often has a higher response rate when it is part of a biochemo cocktail with other chemo drugs. The high dose hasn't worked well enough and there are other treatments with better results and fewer side effects.

My oncologist said there was an IL-2 shop in Dallas at another hospital. Yet, if he had his way, he would send me out of town to get treated by "the best melanoma doctors in the country." They had gotten Interferon approved by the Federal Drug Administration. So I asked their names. He named two doctors from Pittsburgh, Pennsylvania at the University of Pittsburgh. I had to laugh at the irony. Just one week after my dad's funeral, which I had missed, my doctor wanted to transfer me to there to be treated by the same doctors on whom my dad had pinned his hopes. It dawned on me then, if my dad had survived another week, we might have ended up on the same hospital floor.

I found myself hanging on to the verse in 1 Corinthians 10:13, "God is faithful, who will not allow you to be tempted beyond what you are able to bear." I was hoping He had his hand on a pressure relief valve inside of me, since there were moments I thought I was about to burst. I jumped at the chance to go home and be with my family, but I was torn up by the timing issues. I really needed and wanted to be with the Pittsburgh clan. Their love and support had been there all my life, but I often took it for granted. And regrettably, I did not offer much in return, but fortunately, they had short memories as they rallied to my side. Though they put on a brave face, I knew they too were deeply grieving the loss of my dad. I am certain my siblings were heavy with the thought they might soon be burying a brother, and it is one of the hardest tragedies of life, that a mother should outlive a son.

After my plane touched down in Pittsburgh, as it taxied to the gate, it skidded on some ice and got stuck in a huge pile of snow. It took a couple hours to dig us out. Home, sweet home. I was totally frustrated with my first meeting with the Pittsburgh doctor. Since I had no measurable tumors, he said I should be treated with Interferon. I thought my Dallas doctor and he had agreed on the IL-2. I could have taken Interferon in Dallas. He said before receiving any treatment, I would need to be restaged with another PET/CAT scan. We could have set the Pittsburgh scans up immediately from Dallas, so this delayed my treatment another three weeks. The PET results put us back on the IL-2 track anyway, so more precious time had been wasted because of avoidable human errors. The cancer had spread to my right pelvis and to the head and tail of my pancreas. The pancreas is one of the most cancer sensitive of all of the major organs. So this news was very disheartening.

The theory behind IL-2 seemed sound to me. I liked that the treatment worked together with the body's immunities. Interleukins are naturally occurring proteins that trigger a counter attack by the immune system on foreign invaders, called antigens. Cancer cells are not identified as invaders by the immune system's radar, which allows them to multiply freely. So the concept is to flood the system with large quantities of IL-2 proteins to trigger a massive immune reaction and hopefully knock out the cancer. They said IL-2 was effective for a "complete response" about 6% of the time. A complete response means the metastatic melanoma goes away entirely for five years. For advanced Stage IV patients with multiple and "bulky" sites, the odds were much less, but IL-2 was better than doing nothing. I was hoping God wouldn't be working from those statistics anyway.

The plan was for 4 treatment cycles. A cycle included five days of round the clock doses every eight hours. The maximum allowable doses per cycle is 14. There was a one week break between cycles one and two and also between three and four. I would have a two week half time break between cycles two and three. The most serious side effect of IL-2 is fluid built up due to the leaking of fluids from blood capillaries into surrounding tissues. This can cause many side effects, but the most common is renal failure in which the kidneys shut down. If a patient doesn't urinate enough, they are required to skip a dose. So to keep things flowing and manage this side effect, some treatment centers introduce massive amounts of intravenous fluids into the body. The most noticeable side effect of the IL-2 is the flu-like symptoms. You may remember from a high school science class, but fevers and chills are actually not caused by the virus, but by the body's attempts to rid itself of the virus. Turning up the heat, and dropping the temperature are God's strategies to kill viruses. So when massive doses of IL-2 are released intravenously during treatment, the body responds by initiating intense fever and chills.

My first cycle began in early March 2003. At first, it wasn't too hard, but after about 6 doses, I was secretly hoping to not only skip a dose, but skip town. They kept telling me, the more the merrier, so I pushed on. It was like the worst flu I ever had, times three. I would begin to shake off the effects of a dose when the nurse would show up and hang another bag. My skin turned all red and blotchy. My tongue turned white, which they called "thrush", and many of my toenails began turning white. They said that was caused by fungus. My big toenails both eventually fell off. The fever and aches were so intense at times that I began to hallucinate. I was dazed and a very depressing feeling washed over me. I began muttering senseless phrases in a very repetitive manner. I tried to stop but would soon find myself repeating these phrases again. This really bugged me since I felt control of my mind slipping away. I tried to read my Bible, but sometimes I just lay there crying out to God, and often I just lay there crying. I was frustrated with myself because of my inability to sense God or draw comfort from Him. I realized through this fog that the Lord was teaching me something. I had always thought and taught it was our responsibility to depend on God, regardless of our circumstances. If we don't hang on, then it's our fault, too bad, so sad, because this is the way God works. This experience transformed my theology forever. He spoke to me, not audibly, but in my spirit, that though I was losing my grip, what was important was that He had a grip on me. He was my Stronghold! I experienced the reality of Psalm 9:9, "The LORD also will be a stronghold for the oppressed, a stronghold in times of trouble." I have seen the same type of despair and frustration in the eyes of other seriously ill people. They can't seem to get a grip or hang on to the Lord. He seems a million miles away. What should they do? Before the cancer experience, I might have said, "You need to read your Bible more." Now I say, "If you're losing your grip, don't worry. Remember, He's got a hold on you, and He will not let you go."

I was glad my siblings in Pittsburgh took turns staying overnight with me in the hospital. They took care of all the little things and helped me stay focused. I also found myself missing the spiritual input and church services of my congregation back in Dallas. But when I returned to Dallas, I began really missing my Pittsburgh family. I concluded I needed them all. I never saw myself as needing people that much. So once again I cursed the distance between the two groups of people I loved and needed most.

About half way through the first week of IL-2, I got a visit from a dear relative. She began her career as a nurse but became a top regional administrator in a Pittsburgh area hospital system. After her visit, the hospital staff became extremely attentive to me. One nurse gave me a 20 minute massage to warm me up. I was worried other patients might be neglected. I found out later my relative had marked my chart "VIP." One day a nurse cornered one of my sisters in the hall. She wanted to know, "Who is he?" My sister responded, "I can't tell you." The added intrigue made the staff even more curious and attentive. Frankly though, being a VIP on the chemo floor was like having a friendly puppy blow into your arms while being sucked up in the vortex of a tornado. It was nice, but didn't really solve my problem. I knew the Lord was trying to encourage me though, so I received the extra care with gladness. You know, friends in high places.

After the 11th dose of IL-2, my kidneys began to seize up. When I missed two doses in a row, they declared an end to my first cycle and sent me home. I was glad to have managed 11 of 14 of the doses. Doctors, family, friends and church were all very pleased. Privately, I was concerned expectations were being set too high. I knew my body had grown more resistant with each dose.

Chapter Eleven

~~~

A Time for Surrender

*Ecclesiastes 3:1, 6 - There is an appointed time for every-
thing. And there is a time for every event under heaven— a
time to give up.*

During the one week break between IL-2 cycles, I reconnected
with some of my Pittsburgh high school buddies. These guys
are life long friends. They rallied alongside me, despite the fact I
hadn't kept in very good contact over the years. One night, I could
tell they let me win their money in a poker game. Another night
we went out for wings. I was having trouble eating, so I ordered a
milkshake. The waiter said sorry, but they didn't serve milkshakes.
One of my friends said, "You do now. You have milk, and you have
ice cream. Now go get him a milkshake." After drinking most of it,
we left the restaurant abruptly when I began feeling pretty ragged.
I threw up in the parking lot between some cars, which probably
didn't help the cause of milkshakes being added to the menu. My
pancreas was really shutting down. It began to hurt all the time, not
just when I ate. The pancreas is not one of those optional organs.
When pancreatic ducts are sealed off, digestive enzymes designed to
break down fats and carbs will begin to digest the pancreas itself.

On the first day of my second cycle of IL-2, the 2003 invasion
of Iraq kicked off during my first dose. The irony was thick to me.
The theme song for CNN's coverage reverberated throughout the

hospital. I called it "the war tune." It was intense for all Americans to view the constant explosions while worrying about our troops and civilians. I probably shouldn't have been watching the coverage 24/7, but like many Americans, I couldn't stop. I understood why the nurses were distracted too. They kept asking me for updates. When folks called to check on my condition, they eventually brought up the war. Granted, it was kind of a big deal, but I admit I had some resentment about the timing. It really increased my sense of isolation. I began yelling internally, "Hello, I am slowly being tortured to death up here in this hospital bed, does anybody really care?" I imagined slipping away with an obligatory two day mention on the obituary page, which in those days no one was reading. They were all watching the war on TV. And the war tune blared on.

I hesitate to share how I felt about my second cycle of IL-2. I think too many people pass on hard treatments like IL-2 and chemo because of the horror stories. But people need to know; sometimes these stories have a very happy ending. So here goes... My second IL-2 cycle was a four day nightmare, but I called it a daymare. With nightmares, you wake up and realize it is not really happening. Every negative symptom from the first cycle was magnified. The shakes and fevers were more intense. The hallucinations were longer and more frequent, and senseless repetitive phrases constantly droned on in my mind. One night, my shivering was so intense that my bed began shimmying across the floor. They had to lock down the wheels. Several times during the cycle the doctors required me to skip a dose to give my kidneys time to recover. The tipping point for me was on day four when my heart began racing at a rate that was unacceptable to me. My pulse was over 160, as if I had just sprinted in a 100 yard dash, but it lasted for 45 minutes. Frankly that really scared me, especially since one side effect of high dose IL-2 is heart failure. I had had enough. I pulled the plug on the treatment. "Yes, I'm sure!" They may have gotten one of two more doses into me, but I was sure I might die if I got one more drop of the stuff. Nurses and doctors and med students began filing into my room with long faces. "I heard you want to stop. That's too bad." I felt like saying, "No actually I just want to switch places with you." They released me and said they would see me in a couple weeks for the next cycle.

I told them I wasn't so sure about returning. I didn't believe the IL-2 was working, because the pain in my pancreas was still increasing. I missed my wife and kids and church and wanted to go back home to Dallas. I thought if I decided to get more IL-2, I could connect with the IL-2 oncologist in Dallas.

The day after my release, during a Sunday church service in Pittsburgh, I had a sudden attack of pancreatitis, like a knitting needle was being jabbed into my side. I left the service and went back to my mom's house where I had been staying. I felt so bad for her. She had just endured her husband's sickness and death, now her son was writhing on her couch, ravaged by the same disease. We called my doctors and they told me to go back to the emergency room at the same hospital. I swallowed six or seven Advils which didn't even dent the pain. Now I am not sure why they made a cancer patient wait for five hours in that crowded emergency room. They refused my request of "something for the pain" because I had not been admitted and no doctor had seen me. Obviously, the VIP list had not been posted down in the ER. At least the NCAA basketball playoffs were on. When they finally found a room for me, it was the same room where I had my IL-2 treatments. To me, that felt like a cruel joke. I was utterly deflated to be back inside those four walls, which instantly closed in on me again. Doctors gave me some pain meds, which helped to calm me down. I just stopped eating though. The drugs were not strong enough to stop the pain of my pancreas trying to break down food. My wife overheard my doctor and med students conversing in the hall. They were discussing alcohol abuse as a possible cause of my pancreatitis. By this time, they knew I was a preacher. When one tried to rule out alcohol abuse on the basis of my occupation, another said, "That doesn't mean anything. You should see my priest, he drinks like a fish." So they came into my room and began quizzing me about my alcohol intake. I told them the truth; I had only a drink or two per year since my first year of college. Unconvinced, one med student promised me confidentiality out of sensitivity to my profession. I eventually said, "C'mon, look at my scans, I have tumors on both ends of my pancreas growing towards the middle. I have a huge mass at the tail of my pancreas which is six inches by three inches. Think that might cause a little pain?" I watch doctor shows on TV. I know people can drop through the proverbial cracks because of bad assumptions, but this was not one of medicine's finer moments.

The doctor told me I could not be released until I could eat a liquid diet without pain. So for three days I tried to eat Jell-O and soup, but the pain only worsened. To this point, I had been a relatively cooperative patient, but I was getting fussier by the hour. I figured they probably wanted to get rid of me as much as I wanted to go. Matters came to a head one day when I made yet another cranky appeal for release. The doctor seemed ready for me this time. He barked back, "Look, you came all the way from Dallas to get treatment here because you thought we know what we are doing. So calm down, because I refuse to release you until you can eat."

I was embarrassed I had driven the doctor to holler at me. I felt like I had let God down, but mostly I was disappointed in myself. I had taught the passage in James 1:2 so often over the years: "Count it all joy when you encounter various trials." The Lord can give us strength to handle anything. We should let our light shine during tough times and be a good testimony. Of course, all of that is easy to teach. Ironically though, the doctor's speech actually slapped me out of the self-pity funk. I began to seek a different release, in that place which had thus far eluded me – true surrender. I meditated on a strangely liberating passage in Habakkuk 3:17-19,

> *Though the fig tree should not blossom and there be no fruit on the vines, though the yield of the olive tree should fail and the fields produce no food, though the flock should be cut off from the fold and there be no cattle in the stalls, yet I will exult in the LORD, I will rejoice in the God of my salvation. The Lord GOD is my strength, and He has made my feet like hinds' feet, and makes me walk on my high places.*

The flow of earthly blessings in my life had stopped, but I still had my God. He is always good and His love will always be enough. Within 8 hours, another doctor took over as head of the floor. I was still not eating, but he released me on the promise I would pick up treatment with the Interleukin doctor in Dallas. This ongoing wrestling match with the Lord was reflected in my article in the church newsletter in April of 2003. I entitled it simply; "Surrender." No indication yet of sweet surrender, but I was making progress. This is the article:

When you see the word "surrender," what comes to mind? Losing? Giving up? Waving the white flag? It is defined by Danny Webster, "To yield to the power, control, or possession of another upon compulsion or demand." God desires surrender in His children, but the type He seeks includes a glad willingness to undergo struggle or hardship—without the compulsion.

An Example of Surrender

Let's peek in on the apostles Paul and Silas who have just been severely beaten because of their witness for Christ (Acts 16). They are imprisoned in the city jail at Philippi. Instead of complaining and plotting how to get out, they begin "praying and singing praises to God." A great earthquake is sent by a pleased God that levels the prison. They are miraculously freed, yet choose not to disappear into the night. They persuade the jailer not to kill himself, and voluntarily stay under his guard until morning. This act of kindness actually spares the life of the jailer, who would have been put to death for allowing prisoners to escape. They speak the Word to the jailer, and he and his entire household are saved. You see—God's glory was foremost, and their comfort a low priority.

Surrender is voluntarily setting aside personal comfort and agenda for a higher purpose—the glory of God, and the spread of His truth. We live in a cultural climate that stresses indulgence and self-fulfillment. We have thousands of modern conveniences, drugs and equipment that remove discomfort from our lives. "Make your life easier!" and "Why suffer?" are the messages that bombard our souls.

The Need for Surrender

But God stands ready to recruit true followers whose comfort takes a back seat to glorifying Him. I have been called to a physical suffering with cancer that has greatly challenged my comfort levels. I have choices every day to embrace the suffering, or to fuss and complain. Some days I admit I am just kind of numb— not feeling particularly much of anything. Then God reminds me that He has a plan which brings great comfort to me, knowing this suffering is not in vain. Surrender is easier when I know HE dwells inside me and He is ACTIVE. One doesn't have to have a medical condition to practice surrender. We need surrender to live with and love imperfect people at home; to accept that obnoxious co-worker and truly care for his soul; to speak up for Christ despite the jitters. Ironically, it is only through surrender that we find victorious, overcoming living as we yield voluntarily to His plans.

Genuine surrender is usually foisted upon us, and it often comes through a process. My brother once shared a recovery lesson with me. We usually pass through desperation before we find surrender, but the two should not be confused. I was feeling some of both.

Chapter Twelve

~~~

The "Gift" of Cancer

Romans 8:28 - And we know that God causes all things to work together for good to those who love God, to those who are called according to His purpose.

After returning to Dallas, my continuing education class in the school of surrender came in an unexpected way. I had a talk with a sweet friend who was battling Hodgkin's lymphoma. I wanted to trade war stories, but she said something that haunted me. "The Lord is doing so many good things in my life and in the lives of my family and friends. Cancer is such a gift." From my vantage point, the balance of the forty-five minute conversation was eclipsed by the "gift" reference. I was a bit offended and could only think, "Speak for yourself." She had so much faith and optimism that God was going to heal her. She said she had a very treatable disease. She said she had looked up the cancer and acknowledged the statistics were not as promising, but we found passionate agreement on one certainty, God is bigger than any sickness. Ironically, in just a few months, she had moved on to be with the Lord. She was a vivacious, thoughtful and energetic woman. She was truly a gift to me, and I know she was so much more to her family and friends. The impact of her perspective lives on. The conversation proved to be a turning point for my attitude, and for me, the gift of cancer would keep on giving… on this side.

I discovered a powerful book on surrender and finding purpose in trials, called "Streams in the Desert", compiled by Elizabeth Cowman. I devoured the readings. I began to find the encouragement which Paul spoke of when he wrote 2 Corinthians 4:16, "Therefore we do not lose heart, but though our outer man is decaying, yet our inner man is being renewed day by day." I was profoundly aware of the decay. Between the stomach surgery and pancreatitis my body was wasting away. I could eat very little and began losing strength and weight. I had already lost 30 pounds and would eventually lose about 30 more. Not to be too dramatic, I did have a few pounds to spare. Despite the loss of energy, I longed to reengage with my church. I decided to try to preach on Sunday, April 6 of 2003. I gave a report on the things the Lord had been teaching me – "Cancer Lessons." After the service, as I stepped on to my front porch, I felt something pop in my leg. Our dear family friend caught me before I fell. Throughout the entire ordeal, this friend had been holding me and the family up in one way or another. She cooked, cleaned, shuttled, prayed, encouraged, communicated, ran interference – you name it – she was there for us. What a blessing the Lord had provided. Sometimes He grips us through human hands. We discovered that melanoma had spread to lymph nodes in my pelvis and grown from front to the back of my pelvis, invading my ischium bone, one of the sitting bones. The popping noise was the ischium fracturing. I got some crutches and began using them constantly. Trying to lighten things up, someone at church said, "Don't you think you're getting enough attention around here that you need to start limping around on crutches?" I usually try not to take myself too seriously and I've delivered my share of clunker jokes, but the comment really twisted me the wrong way. I think I felt guilty for getting a lot of attention. Alas, another opportunity to surrender. I decided to forgive and move on.

As time passed, I realized what my friend meant about cancer being a gift. I heard from people I hadn't seen or talked to for years. Many relationships were rekindled in beautiful ways. Several people who had left our church unhappy for various reasons visited me to apologize about the way they had treated me. I trust they did not regret apologizing when I didn't die. Eventually, the Lord managed to get a better grip on me. This is the newsletter article which I wrote for our church in June of 2003, entitled "Center Point":

There he is again with that same look on his face. It's the valet guy at the chemo center. The first day he helped me out of the car he said "Wow, this is really cramping your style." I assumed he was thinking that I am young and active and full of plans and this was the last place I wanted to be. He was right. Last week he tells me, "Now go up there and tell those doctors and nurses that you have more important things to be doing." I know he feels for me, yet he continually raises the question that I cannot shake. Why?

Things I loved and enjoyed have been tabled. I've missed many events and moments with my kids. No playing basketball, fishing, barbecuing, no Bible studies with my high school Ironmen group. No preaching or singing on Sunday mornings. This is all very hard for me. I guess I found so much purpose and refreshment in those things.

On the other hand, I see some wonderful blessings in the midst. My relationship with my wife is better than ever. We have grown close and knitted together while seeking hope and encouragement from God and each other. I have renewed old acquaintances and been brought to tears by encouragement and prayers from great friends and even from total strangers.

The Center of His Will

But ultimately I don't evaluate this season in my life by comparing gains and losses. The foundation remains that God has me in this spot for His purpose. When I gave Him my life some 22 years ago, I meant it. "Do with me what you will, God. I trust you will not give me more than I can handle with your strength." So I take great delight in this alone; I am smack dab in the center of His will. Clarity will come later. Lights will turn on and all will make perfect sense.

Wiggling Away from Center

There is an overarching passion in the human heart—we prefer things easy and comfortable. Yet we are continually hand-cuffed, criss-crossed and disappointed by the realities of life. Jesus appeared to Saul, who would become Paul the apostle, and told him to "quit kicking against the goads." The expression comes from a horse which kicks back against its master's attempts to steer and motivate him. God wanted Paul to settle into His plan for his life.

It is easy to kick against the goads. Maybe your marriage is not what you want it to be. The boss undervalues and under-pays you. You see character flaws in your children that deeply concern you. You feel your life is slipping by and you haven't even come close to meeting your potential. So we choose depression, frustration, fussing and complaining. We fight and quarrel and manipulate to try to smooth our path. Or we may just kind of check out and go through the motions.

Aim for the Center

That is no way for God's children to live. We are more than conquerors. We are His pride and joy and He gives everything we need to not only survive, but to thrive in any situation. The center of God's will is crowded with troubles. Don't deny them or ignore them, but don't focus on them either. Turn your eyes to the One who overcomes trouble and let Him lift your spirits and give you joy in the storms and wisdom to handle the struggles. What more important thing could we be doing?

There is an old Christian saying, "Sometimes He calms the storm, and sometimes He calms the child." My question was, "Does the child sometimes get to pick?"

Chapter Thirteen

~~~

Brink of Death

Philippians 2:21 – For to me, to live is Christ and to die is gain.

We had been frantically researching trials and vaccines on the internet and by phone. A Dallas researcher had reportedly made some serious strides against melanoma. He was isolating and multiplying a patient's own dendretic, or cancer-killing cells, to seek out and eliminate melanoma. We had to qualify for the trial, so we met with him in early April. It was quickly apparent that I was not deemed a good candidate. My case was too advanced. I learned a lot about these promising new trials that receive a lot of hype in the media. I am not being critical, because these researchers work very hard and are very smart, but progress against late stage melanoma is slow. These studies usually screen out advanced cases, which greatly skew the results. The trial doctor's nurse took Terri aside, and told her in a matter of fact fashion, "When the melanoma gets to their pancreas, they go really fast." The doctor told me, "You have a raging fire that needs to be calmed down some other way, like through chemo, and then you should come back." This is not what you want to hear from a fireman when he drives up and your house is ablaze.

My first appointment with my new Dallas oncologist was very hopeful. I went to him because he was the only doctor in Dallas able to treat metastatic melanoma with IL-2. He was also highly recommended by our melanoma mentor, a man whose wife had melanoma for years. Her melanoma originated in her eye. Many times he patiently answered all of our questions and gave several medical tips the Lord ultimately used to save my life. From the start, my new oncologist was very engaged and concerned. He wanted to hospitalize me immediately, which didn't go over well with me. He ordered an MRI on my hip and leg, but he was most concerned about my lack of food intake. I told him it was too painful to eat. He said, "You can't just stop eating. We need to put you on TPN immediately." TPN is Total Parenteral Nutrition, a milky fluid given by intravenous drip to provide nutrition. I called it a milk shake and lived exclusively off TPN for almost four months. Terri was trained on how to operate the pump and hook it to my IV. It took about an hour to "drink" my shake and I would immediately feel my strength increase. I was glad to be under this doctor's care but we wondered why no one had recommended TPN until now. Frankly, I think they hadn't because they thought it would merely prolong the inevitable.

Another PET scan showed more melanoma spreading into my celiac trunk, a branched artery that provides blood to the spleen, liver and stomach. I also developed two new lumps just under my skin above and below my collar bone. They grew to the size of large grapes and in a way served as a monitor for my melanoma. Terri felt the lumps many times a day and was constantly praying them away. At this point everyone was sensing the curtain would soon drop. My brother came down from Pittsburgh and found a place to stay in Dallas. He told me later he thought someone from our immediate family should be with me when I died. I suspected that is why he stayed with no stated departure date, but it was nice to have him around. We watched several Dallas Mavericks NBA playoff games together. My brother-in-law and sister-in-law and her husband came to stay for a few days. They were a big lift to me as well. They boldly agreed to come back as soon as I was well, and they did. At the time, however, I know they had to wonder if their next trip would be for a funeral. I sometimes would look out the window to watch visitors as they walked to their cars. I knew it might be my last glimpse of them on the earth. One relative broke down in tears as he stepped down off the porch. Once some good friends came to visit. They later told me they were all jacked up to encourage me and lay hands on me and pray for my healing. When they saw me, they were stunned by my condition, and it threw them off the plan, wondering if maybe it was my time to go.

I used to breeze by the obituaries in the newspaper. Now, every day I was reading every word on the obit page. I imagined what my obit might say. I pondered how long I would be missed, and how long I would be remembered. I wondered if you could watch your own funeral from heaven. Could a person be disappointed in heaven if their funeral attendance was low? I found myself wishing I could have some "do overs" of a few decisions. I wished I had treated my wife and kids better. She had been so tireless and selfless while taking care of me, which made me feel closer, and guiltier. Most of all, I wished I could have reached more people for Christ. I had this gnawing sense that I was not done with my life's work. It felt like the canvas was being jerked away just as I was learning how to paint.

Chapter Fourteen

~~~

Days to Live

Job 7:3-4 - Nights of trouble are appointed me. When I lie down I say, "When shall I arise?" But the night continues, and I am continually tossing until dawn.

On Easter Sunday, in May of 2003, I was determined to deliver the sermon. Though I felt very weak, my imagination had been stirred by the thought of a miraculous healing. Why not? There are millions of daily miracles occurring all around us. Would it be too difficult to send one my way? I spoke about the new growth of spring and the new babies in the congregation. These are "natural" miracles we tend to take for granted. Of course I spoke of the most significant miracle, the resurrection of Jesus Christ, which was God's trumping of death's grasp on man. Since it is so true, nothing is impossible with God, I encouraged each member of the church to seek a miracle in their own life. My sister was visiting at the time. She had been watching me stagger around the house, and asked if I was crazy to try to preach. Later she said, "How did you do that?" Certainly much supernatural strength had been provided and some human adrenaline was also involved but I paid a hefty price. During the worship leader's closing prayer, I leaned over to Terri and said, "Let's go, now!" As I stumbled to the car, I almost fainted because of the pain in my pancreas. I wondered if the best miracle would be for Him to take me home on the spot. I was writhing and crying as I tried to get situated in the car which was parked right outside of the church. One of the church members had followed us out and was watching me through the lobby window of the church. As soon as I noticed her watching, I pretended not to hurt, but she had already started to break down in tears. I believe she was thinking the obvious, that my miracle had better hurry. As we rode away from the church, I wondered if that was my last sermon.

A few days later I was hospitalized again. I felt like there was a large blockage in my midsection. They ran an MRI and an endoscopy but could find nothing in my digestive tract to account for the pain. They concluded it must be the cancer in my pancreas. The nurses told me whenever my pain grew intense, that they would give me a shot of a painkiller drug called dilaudid. Also called hydromorphone, dilaudid is such a strong opiate that it's closely monitored by the government with triple prescription forms. I found the drug to be an absolute wonder. Ahhhhh! Wow. After a dose, whenever nurses asked how I was doing, I would say, "Pretty darn good actually." But if I hinted there was any pain, off they went to bring more diluadid. I began worrying that I liked the drug a little too much. So I mentioned the concern to a nurse and she said, "Oh don't worry about that, the doctor said to keep you comfortable." Whoa! Wait a minute, what did you just say? I told her the comment sounded like something they say to a terminally ill patient when there is nothing more they can do. They had not given up on me yet, had they? I had not been consulted, or at least notified of this new approach. The nurse extracted herself graciously, realizing that she had let a tiger out of the bag. Soon my oncologist came for a visit. He gently gave me a get-your-things-in-order speech. He finished with, "You have just days to live." I knew I was in really bad shape; still, his timetable caught me off guard. I asked, "You're not saying months, or even weeks, but days?" He said based on his experience, I had just days to live and I should be prepared. He was right to warn me, yet something rose up in me against the prognosis. Since my doctor was a God-fearing Jewish man, I asked him if he held out any hope of a divine turnaround. He said he had been in this situation before, many times, and that though it was not likely that I would recover, it was indeed possible. I didn't set out to give him a hard time, but at this point I was not ready to throw in the towel. I boldly suggested that he might die before me. Again he politely acknowledged the possibility, but denied the likelihood. We did agree he could get hit by a truck as he walked to his car after work. So I flipped the question, and asked if *he* were ready to die. We had a very deep and constructive conversation about Judaism and Christianity which lasted well over an hour. I was concerned about his other patients, but I decided to defer to his timing on ending the discussion. He said he found something very impressive about the way Jesus Christ had impacted history. I interpreted the comment as permission to back up the gospel truck, and I dumped the entire load. He seemed to enjoy the spiritual banter. In fact, later that day on his rounds, he returned to announce he was telling everyone in the hospital about a great conversation he had with a Christian minister. I was delighted for the opportunity to share my faith with a man I now consider a friend.

Still, the doctor's cautions about my life expectancy rattled me. I concluded that in case he was right, I should prepare to die. I called in a good friend who was a leader at our church. I began nailing down preparations for my funeral. I picked the songs and the scripture readings. But I had an overriding request: "Whatever you do, make me look good." I know, tall order.

After hearing my prognosis, I felt like I was in a limbo, hovering between life and death. During the night, as I tried to sleep, I began fretting over what it was like to die. I think maybe it was not so much the fear of death that bothered me, but rather the fear of dying. I knew death was inevitable, but would mine be not only early, but slow, painful and torturous? The possibility of experiencing even more suffering began to short circuit my belief in the goodness and power of God. Then an insidious doubt slipped in. Maybe God was not able or willing to prevent additional pain. The concept somehow took a deep foothold in my mind. Soon waves of doubts flooded my thoughts. I didn't tell anyone about this battle until much later, since I was embarrassed by my lack of faith. Why did God seem so distant? Does He really measure out our trials so they are not too much to handle? I felt like I had long passed the point of being able to bear that level of pain. How do I know for sure there is a heaven anyway? I had never actually seen God and I certainly couldn't feel Him now. Maybe God does not even exist after all.

As I lay dying in the darkened hospital room, raucous laughter from the nurses' station kept disrupting my train of thought. Though it was the night shift, I didn't fault the nurses. I could have asked them to keep it down and they would have been quieter, but I decided to just think and listen. The message was humbling; the world would go on without me. If my heart monitor were to flat line, the nurses would call the coroner, wrap me in a sheet, and say it was a shame since I was not that old. Then they would go back to their laughing. For several nights I lay there, dreading a slow, painful death and listening to the sounds of happiness in the hallway. Those were the dark nights of my soul.

Chapter Fifteen

~~~

Back to Basics

Psalm 19:1-4 - A Psalm of David. The heavens are telling of the glory of God; and their expanse is declaring the work of His hands. Day to day pours forth speech, And night to night reveals knowledge. There is no speech, nor are there words; Their voice is not heard. Their line has gone out through all the earth, and their utterances to the end of the world. In them He has placed a tent for the sun.

I knew I must dig out of the funk, but hard as I tried, I could not. My faith had evaporated when I needed it most. Like a knight without a shield, invisible archers took full advantage of the opening. I cried out to God, uncertain whether He was listening or even there. Then I sensed Him explaining my emotions had overtaken the proofs of His existence and His Word. I needed to stop feeling my way through this struggle and return to focusing on His perspective. He empowered me to fight back. Starting from square one, I began to resist the doubt. The existence of this incredibly complex universe demanded an infinite, eternal Creator. I recalled the days of my youth when my dad took the boys to stay at a fishing cabin in the mountains of Pennsylvania. At night the canopy of stars seemed so close, so bright, almost within arms reach. We would lay on our backs, gazing upward, scanning the sky for shooting stars. There was something magical about those evenings for me. I concluded someone great and good had fashioned the show. During my teen years, I often gazed at my own hand, fascinated by the intricacy of its workings. A pile of gray mush we call a brain could actually send electrical impulses to my hand and fingers to move, point and ball my fingers into a fist. The proof of such remarkable design had left me astonished that anyone could ever doubt there is a God. Now three decades later, while lying on my death bed, I raised up my hand in front of my face to gaze at its workings. Once more I moved and pointed and balled up my fingers into a fist. How could such design have resulted from nothingness and chance? This evidence was like a peg of encouragement pounded into a cliff of doubts. I was getting traction.

My thoughts moved from nature to history. I was reminded that a man named Jesus Christ, who claimed to be the divine Son of God, had entered time and space and delivered an unprecedented impact on human history. Even my Jewish doctor, who was not raised to acknowledge this source of evidence, was thoroughly impressed! For two thousand years, Jesus' teachings have marked and even guided man's philosophy. He revamped our calendar. We divide history into two, B.C. and A.D.; his birth being the pivotal point of the human story. He confirmed His divinity by rising from the dead, an event verified by substantial historical evidence. There were a number of eyewitnesses of the resurrected Christ; several described their encounters in a reliable book we call the New Testament. By standard measures of reliability, such as numbers and similarities of manuscripts, the New Testament stands out among other ancient books such as Homer's Iliad and Odyssey, from which we unquestioningly derive much history. Though the New Testament has been constantly maligned, it has stood the test of time. Many have attempted to snuff out these eyewitness accounts of Jesus' life, just as they managed to silence the authors themselves. Critics have scoffed at the book's ability to hold up under enlightened scrutiny. I recalled reading that in 1778 the French philosopher, Voltaire, infamously predicted, "One hundred years from my day there will not be a Bible in the earth except one that is looked upon by an antiquarian curiosity seeker." Clearly, Voltaire was neither a prophet nor as smart as he thought. The Bible remains the best selling book every year since such records have been kept. Some estimate the Bible has sold six billion copies. My confidence began returning.

As a love letter and treasure map from our Creator, the New Testament is not only trustworthy, it is intensely personal. Within its pages is a bold declaration of unconditional love which the Creator has for us. The Father ultimately proved this love in real time by sending His Son to die in my place. I have experienced this love personally many times in the form of unexplainable blessings, answered prayers and internal peace. Through the freedom I found through a relationship with Jesus Christ, I was set free from enslaving sins and excesses of my youth - drugs, alcohol abuse and tobacco. In the Bible, this same Jesus who had personally proven His existence and presence many times had promised eternal life; that all who believe in Him will be forever with Him in heaven. In John 14:1-3, He promised,

"Do not let your heart be troubled; believe in God, believe also in Me. In My Father's house are many dwelling places; if it were not so, I would have told you; for I go to prepare a place for you. If I go and prepare a place for you, I will come again and receive you to Myself, that where I am, there you may be also."

So I renewed my stand, that I had already received His offer by faith. Deep assurances of God's love began steadying my shaky soul. The warming, relaxing sense of His Presence returned. His closeness was all I really needed and a new type of faith welled up within me. A faith I had never experienced or even needed before. It was a faith that brought confidence in the face of even a slow, painful kind of death. He held me up until I regained my footing. It dawned on me once again, that though I had lost my grip, He had a grip on me. My Stronghold.

Chapter Sixteen

~~~

To Live Or Not To Live

Philippians 2:21-25 - For to me, to live is Christ and to die is gain. But if I am to live on in the flesh, this will mean fruitful labor for me; and I do not know which to choose. But I am hard-pressed from both directions, having the desire to depart and be with Christ, for that is very much better; yet to remain on in the flesh is more necessary for your sake. Convinced of this, I know that I will remain and continue with you all for your progress and joy in the faith.

As the Lord rebuilt my faith, my emotional pendulum swung a whole new direction. During the stay in the hospital which lasted until the first week of April 2003, I began marveling at a verse which seemed to jump off the page at me. "For to me, to live is Christ and to die is gain" (Philippians 2:21). I was now very ready to die, maybe too ready. I began asking, even begging the Lord to take me home. I now totally understand why people refuse treatment at the end of their lives. I just wanted relief. I was so tired. As the saying goes, I had used up all my sick days, so I decided to call in dead. Terri wanted me to live on though. She believed the Lord had spoken previously to her that I would not die. Yet when she saw how much I was struggling, she decided not to cling to me. She "released" the Lord from what she believed was His clear promise to her and decided to have it out with Him later. She likened it to

Abraham letting go of the promise of Isaac when he was called to sacrifice Isaac.

As the news of my sentiment spread quickly among friends and the church, there was an unexpected reaction. One good friend, called and said, "What's this I hear about you wanting to die. Forget about that. We want you and need you here. Your kids need you here and Terri needs you here. You are going to be fine, so snap out of this." She has always been a great friend and said it with a good spirit. At the time, however, I was offended. I felt she was clueless as to my situation. I was being tortured and I was crying "Uncle." Let her get in the ring for a few rounds. I began to soften though as the Lord opened up 2 Corinthians 4:17 to me; "For momentary, light affliction is producing for us an eternal weight of glory far beyond all comparison." I had been comparing this pain-filled time period with my life before the cancer. So it was not surprising that I wanted to check out. Instead, I needed to compare my present sufferings to the awesome weight of the glory of God to be revealed in the next life. Paul was right; our suffering has a bearable lightness when placed in front of the backdrop of ultimate bliss. My friend was right too and the Lord used her exhortation to turn my heart.

I dove into the verses that follow Philippians 2:21. There Paul considers the impact on others of both his departure and his continuing to live.

Philippians 2:22-25 - But if I am to live on in the flesh, this will mean fruitful labor for me; and I do not know which to choose. But I am hard-pressed from both directions, having the desire to depart and be with Christ, for that is very much better; yet to remain on in the flesh is more necessary for your sake. Convinced of this, I know that I will remain and continue with you all for your progress and joy in the faith.

I began to feel a strong tug that God Himself wanted me to fight to stay. I knew the advantages of growing old with Terri. I loved her and she needed help raising our kids. The church could find another pastor; still, I knew I could benefit them. Plus, this lost world could surely use another worker to build bridges to the only hope of salvation, the Savior, Jesus. I would have all eternity to heal up and enjoy the Lord. Now was the time to make my life count and to labor for the sake of others. Heaven could wait. So I began to fight as hard as I could to stay alive.

I realize my take on these scriptures could be unsettling to some. Am I saying we always have the choice to live or die, and the Lord is bound to our choice? Not at all. The Lord has our days numbered and He holds the key to our life span. I do believe, however, that God can instill a fighting faith to live in the face of imminent death. As He did with Paul, He implants the desire to fulfill it. On the flip side of this coin, I have been at the bedsides of extremely ill people who wish to refuse treatment. I have always affirmed that decision. Sometimes people have asked me to help change someone's decision to stop treatment and I have declined. I assume the Lord is leading them too, and that He wants to bring them home sooner than later. Isaiah 57:1 says, "The righteous man perishes, and no man takes it to heart; And devout men are taken away, while no one understands. For the righteous man is taken away from evil." In Psalm 116, the psalmist reports that he was near death, but he cried out for his life and God rescued him. In Psalm 116:9, he writes, "I shall walk before the LORD in the land of the living." Yet a few verses later in verse 15, he presents the other side of this life or death question: "Precious in the sight of the LORD is the death of His godly ones." Wow. This is another way to think about the "premature" death of a loved one. Sometimes God decides He can't wait any longer to bring a person to their ultimate home. The bottom line is the Lord can be glorified in either the life or death of His chosen ones.

Of course, many have passed away who had an unshakeable desire to live. Consider my dad for example. He told me the night before he passed away that he would soon begin a breakthrough melanoma trial which he was convinced would knock out his cancer. If mind over matter and human determination were the only requisites for staying alive, he would definitely be with us today. Then there is the non-survivor who was convinced God had spoken that he was already healed. I have known such people who confidently quoted Bible verses claiming their healing, but instead they were called home. I have to be frank here. When God made a prediction to someone in the Bible, it came to pass. If the event did not transpire, God never promised it in the first place. So I believe that just as there can be a false optimism rooted in positive thinking, there can be spiritually-based false optimism. Both must be distinguished from God-implanted faith that results in healing. You ask, how does one tell the difference? I cannot. In time we will all know. In the meantime, I encourage people to study and pray hard and follow their heart and leave the ultimate outcome to the Lord.

Some survivors scoff at the suggestion that God cured them. Once a student at Stanford asked Lance Armstrong how his belief in God helped him as a cancer patient. Lance replied, "Everyone should believe in something, and I believed in surgery, chemotherapy and my doctors." I agree with Lance, we must believe in something. Yet I ask, "Where does a doctor's intelligence and skills come from?" Fortunately for all of us, God is gracious despite our ungratefulness. In the end, I think we will not have airtight explanations for all of these dilemmas. I suppose that is where faith takes over, prodding us to new levels of trust. I think the tension should humble us at our lack of ultimate wisdom, not anger us at the Lord.

Chapter Seventeen

~~~

What Is Thy Will?

Matthew 6:10 - Your kingdom come. Your will be done, on earth as it is in heaven.

My new found determination "to stick around" was triggered at the end of April 2003. During the next month, Terri and I devoured the scriptures together, studying all of the Bible verses on physical healing. Terri definitely had a head start in this department. While I was adjusting to the fact that I even had cancer, she had been working on landing a healing. Now this was not the first time I studied this topic, but as you might imagine my interest level had increased. Though I didn't want to read my preferences into the scriptures, I admit I was hoping to find guarantees that God would heal me. Divine healing is a controversial topic among Bible students today. Like other biblical controversies, the folks who holler loudest are often found at the extremes, but the truth often lies somewhere in the middle. I think the first step in understanding the Bible is to gather and analyze all of the teaching and narratives on a topic and only then form an overall interpretation. Imbalance happens most often when we "cherry pick" verses on a topic. Even so, it is not easy determining how much weight to give any single passage or set of passages. To thoroughly discuss divine healing, a full length book would be necessary, but for this book I have summarized a few of my basic conclusions.

1) During Jesus' time on earth, He spent a lot of His time healing and alleviating suffering. There is no record of Him ever turning someone away who wanted physical healing. Matthew 4:24 says, "And they brought to Him all who were ill, those suffering with various diseases and pains, demoniacs, epileptics, paralytics; and He healed them." There were other occasions when Gospel writers stressed the point that He healed *all* who pursued Him (Matthew 8:16; Luke 4:40). Sometimes we fail to pursue divine healing because we determine in advance that God probably won't answer in the affirmative. We can become overwhelmed by human statistical probabilities. The epistle of James explains that sometimes we are not answered because we never ask. "We have not because we ask not" (James 3:2). Another mistake we can make is to turn to doctors alone. Consider King Asa's premature demise in 2 Chronicles 16:12-13. "In the thirty-ninth year of his reign Asa became diseased in his feet. His disease was severe, yet even in his disease he did not seek the LORD, but the physicians. So Asa slept with his fathers, having died in the forty-first year of his reign." Clearly, the scriptures present doctors' powers as limited, especially in Mark 5:26. "She had endured much at the hands of many physicians, and had spent all that she had and was not helped at all, but rather had grown worse." Been there. By all means, we should definitely use doctors, since God uses them so often. We should also bang on the doors of heaven for our healing. It is not a case of either/or but both/and.

2) Jesus wants us to believe in His ability to heal. In Matthew 9:28-29, He said, "Do you believe that I am able to do this?" They said to Him, "Yes, Lord." Then He touched their eyes, saying, "It shall be done to you according to your faith."

3) Jesus also wants us to believe in His general willingness to heal. 3 John 1:2 states God's general desire that we remain in good health; "Beloved, I pray that in all respects you may prosper and be in good health, just as your soul prospers."

4) Our unbelief can limit the frequency of divine healings. Speaking of Jesus' healing activity in His hometown, Mark laments

in 6:5-6, "And He could do no miracle there except that He laid His hands on a few sick people and healed them. And He wondered at their unbelief." Are we limiting God's miracles today by our unbelief? Maybe there are so few reported healings in some faith communities because they consider bold faith to be presumptuous. It is clear this cycle could be self-fulfilling. If leaders discourage bold faith, we witness fewer miracles. Then those same leaders point to the scarcity of healings as proof that "God doesn't work that way any more."

5) Some cite Isaiah 53:5 as an absolute guaranteed promise of physical healing: "By His stripes we are healed." They argue that just as Christ suffered death on the cross to take away our sin, so He also suffered bodily in the form of scourgings and beatings to take away our physical suffering. Since eternal salvation is promised and absolutely guaranteed by His death in Isaiah 53, then the promise of divine healing from the very same passage should be guaranteed as well. Some explain away this tension by categorizing the type of healing in Isaiah 53:5 as spiritual and not physical. Mark 8:16-17 settles any dispute by establishing a clear linkage for physical healing in Isaiah 53. "When evening came, they brought to Him many who were demon-possessed; and He cast out the spirits with a word, and healed all who were ill. This was to fulfill what was spoken through Isaiah the prophet: 'He Himself took our infirmities and carried away our diseases.'"

So turning to Isaiah 53 as a promise made sense to me and I began claiming this verse for my physical healing. I must have recited it well over 100 times a day for three months and claimed it as true for me. Was claiming this promise in this manner part of the "reason" God spared my life?

6) Jesus taught that whenever we pray, we should pray with bold faith. Praying for healing is no exception. On several occasions He taught this principle. One such example is in Mark 11:22-24; "Have faith in God. Truly I say to you, whoever says to this mountain, 'Be taken up and cast into the sea,' and does not doubt in his heart, but believes that what he says is going to happen, it will be granted

him. Therefore I say to you, all things for which you pray and ask, believe that you have received them, and they will be granted you." So the typical prayer of every follower of Christ should be full of expressions of thanks that the prayer has already been answered in the affirmative. This manner of praying is not at all the type of faith that is routinely practiced in many circles in the church today. This is not only a lack of faith, it is also a form of rebellion, since it ignores Jesus' clear teaching. Trust me, I am not innocent in this matter either. Should we not all seek to grow in this area?

In his epistle, James commands that we pray for divine healing with faith. In 5:14-18,

> "Is anyone among you sick? Then he must call for the elders of the church and they are to pray over him, anointing him with oil in the name of the Lord; and the prayer offered in faith will restore the one who is sick, and the Lord will raise him up, and if he has committed sins, they will be forgiven him. Therefore, confess your sins to one another, and pray for one another so that you may be healed. The effective prayer of a righteous man can accomplish much. Elijah was a man with a nature like ours, and he prayed earnestly that it would not rain, and it did not rain on the earth for three years and six months. Then he prayed again, and the sky poured rain and the earth produced its fruit."

Previously in his epistle, James defined what he meant by praying with faith in James 1:5-8.

> But if any of you lacks wisdom, let him ask of God, who gives to all generously and without reproach, and it will be given to him. But he must ask in faith without any doubting, for the one who doubts is like the surf of the sea, driven and tossed by the wind. For that man ought not to expect that he will receive anything from the Lord, being a double-minded man, unstable in all his ways.

In this context, praying with faith means believing that once we ask, God will automatically provide the wisdom. If one doubts that God will give the wisdom, they should not expect to receive anything from God. In other words, wisdom is guaranteed. So, we should apply this description of praying with faith to the elders' prayers for healing in James 5. Elders and all others should pray believing we have already received healing once we ask. If we doubt, we should not expect to receive. Jesus wondered aloud during His time on earth whether faith would die out over the centuries. In Luke 18:8, "When the Son of Man comes, will He find faith on the earth?" I decided if I was to be in error in how I prayed for my healing, I would rather err on the side of imitating those with bold faith.

7) When Jesus concluded His requests in the Garden of Gethsemane with the phrase, "... But not My will, but Thy will be done," He was not forever establishing a caveat to tack on to the end of all of our prayers. A close reading of this fascinating exchange reveals that Jesus was not at all trying to discern God's will in this instance. He in fact already knew God's perfect will. His Father had asked Him to be tortured to death, and to take on the sin of the world to boot. So Jesus, who obviously had some serious misgivings about the plan, was attempting to change God's revealed will! At the last minute, He was passionately appealing for a Plan B. So this event is not a good example of how we should typically pray, unless of course we are absolutely certain of God's will on the matter of our healing and seeking to change that will in one way or another.

8) Jesus expected His disciples to have strong enough faith to heal other's sickenesses. He was agitated when His disciples could not heal a demon-possessed boy. In Matthew 17:17-21,

> And Jesus answered and said, "You unbelieving and perverted generation, how long shall I be with you? How long shall I put up with you? Bring him here to Me." And Jesus rebuked him, and the demon came out of him, and the boy was cured at once. Then the disciples came to Jesus privately and said, "Why could we not drive it out?" And He said to them,

"Because of the littleness of your faith; for truly I say to you, if you have faith the size of a mustard seed, you will say to this mountain, 'Move from here to there,' and it will move; and nothing will be impossible to you. But this kind does not go out except by prayer and fasting."

Jesus taught that faith must be exercised to grow and He certainly expects us to have strong faith. Though weak faith can hamper results, we should keep in mind our faith need not be perfect. One father worried his faith was too weak for his son's healing. Jesus had said, "All things are possible to him who believes." The man confessed, "I believe. Help my unbelief," and in the end, he received the healing for his son, despite his doubts (Mark 9:23-24).

9) Jesus intended all generations of His followers to lay hands on the sick for physical healing. In Mark 16:15-18, He speaks of answering healing prayers of first century Christians, and the prayers of subsequent generations as well. "These signs will accompany those who have believed: in My name they will cast out demons, they will speak with new tongues; they will pick up serpents, and if they drink any deadly poison, it will not hurt them; they will lay hands on the sick, and they will recover."

In Acts 2:20, Peter states that supernatural gifts, including divine healing, would be in operation until the coming of the "end times" or "Last Days." The period of these gifts would last, "Before (or until) the great and glorious day of the Lord shall come." The Day of the Lord is a technical term in the scripture which refers to the final tribulation period before the Second Coming of Jesus. So, supernatural expressions of His power through His followers should be expected until that day.

10) There are some biblical caveats on healing. There are exceptions in the New Testament epistles to the general rule that the Lord always healed everyone who sought healing. (The epistles are the letters of Paul and others, and are to be distinguished from the gospels of Matthew, Mark, Luke and John). To me, these exceptions lead to the undeniable conclusion that there is not an absolute

guarantee of physical healing in the Bible. Through denying some requests for healing, the Lord introduced a crucial principle in the lives of His children, which some have called "a higher purpose." One of the clearest examples is Paul's "thorn in the flesh," which he described at length in 2 Corinthians 12. Paul was not referring to a literal thorn, but rather an irritating set of trials which included whippings, beatings, stonings and jailings. Paul asked the Lord three times to remove this thorn, but God did not, telling Paul instead that His grace would enable him to cope and stay humble. In Paul's list of trials, he did not include his struggle with a serious and chronic eye problem, but he explains how this sickness brought about his initial presentation of the good news to the Galatians (Galatians 4:12-16). Evidently, Paul had traveled to the Galatian region not to plant a church, but to get treatment for his eyes. His weakness brought about a strong emotional and spiritual connection with the Galatians, even though that bond faded with time.

> "I beg of you, brethren, become as I am, for I also have become as you are. You have done me no wrong; but you know that it was because of a bodily illness that I preached the gospel to you the first time; and that which was a trial to you in my bodily condition you did not despise or loathe, but you received me as an angel of God, as Christ Jesus Himself. Where then is that sense of blessing you had? For I bear you witness that, if possible, you would have plucked out your eyes and given them to me. So have I become your enemy by telling you the truth?"

One might paraphrase Paul's appeal this way: *"Even though my eye problem was really gross, you did not turn away from me, but were drawn with compassion towards me in seeing me as God's mouthpiece for the message of Jesus. You would have done anything to help me, including becoming an eye donor. So what happened? I would love to rekindle that bond."* We all know that physical suffering has a powerful capacity to soften the human heart, bonding people to God and each other. Like my friend said, sickness or cancer can be a "gift." I have often observed His higher purposes at work to mend and rekindle relationships both in my life and in the lives of others. He also uses sickness as a wakeup call. Like a mother turning her child's face to hers, He knows how to get our attention.

Despite Paul's clear teaching on the way God uses suffering, some in the church consider physical suffering to be pointless and avoidable. And most tragically, some consider an unhealed sickness to be evidence of a lack of faith. They claim that God never wants us to be sick for even a moment. So sick people beat themselves up, or are beaten up by others, because of their doubting. Like Job's friends who failed to understand God's higher purposes, we can compound the pain of the sick. I once heard a great story that might help us come to grips with the foolishness of such teaching.

Once a blind woman sought the counsel of a wise, grandfatherly pastor. Through tears she said, "Pastor, I was born blind, and I've been blind all my life. I don't mind being blind but I have some well meaning friends who tell me that if I had more faith I could be healed."

The pastor asked her, "Tell me, do you carry one of those canes to walk around?"

"Yes I do," she replied.

"Then," he said, "The next time someone says that to you, whack them over the head with the cane. Then tell them, 'If you had more faith, that wouldn't hurt!'"

11) Sometimes God's highest purpose includes the premature death of one of His children. We need to remember, God sees death from an entirely different perspective than us. While we are reeling from loss, He is experiencing a delightful reunion. In Psalm 116, an appeal to the Lord to be rescued from premature death also adds, "Precious in the sight of the LORD is the death of His godly ones." Sometimes God can't wait to reveal His face to a chosen one. Isaiah 57:1-2 adds the idea that He may in fact be doing a person a huge favor by sparing them from the evils of this life or perhaps some specific evil; "The righteous man perishes, and no man takes it to heart; and devout men are taken away, while no one understands. For the righteous man is taken away from evil, he enters into peace."

Though incredibly painful for us, there are compelling reasons the Lord takes a loved one early.

So to draw these concepts together, I believe we should pray boldly and claim healing when we are ill. This type of faith pleased and impressed Jesus when He walked the earth. There is no convincing reason to believe He has changed. He commanded us to pray with faith believing we have what we are asking. Though this type of faith does not guarantee physical healing, we would probably receive more miracles if we prayed with faith. If the Lord does not answer our bold prayers of faith, we can trust He has a Higher Purpose that He is working out for His glory. Such purposes are after all, more important than our comfort, or our earthly existence.

During my fight to stay alive, I became convinced I needed to claim healing and believe God had already healed me. Some people were uncomfortable with this theology, but I noticed people don't like to debate people who have cancer. Terri believed the Lord had spoken to her that He was indeed going to heal me. So she had additional cause to pray boldly. She was not shy about sharing this, especially at our church. I had to chuckle at times when I saw my bride in full prayer combat mode. A couple of church folks timidly tried to prepare Terri for the possibility of my death. They would preface prayers for my healing with the phrase, "Lord, if it be Thy will …" So before a few of our prayer meetings when the elders would anoint me and lay hands on me as prescribed in James 5, she would quiz each of them as to how they were about to pray. Once she asked some folks and any elders to pass on praying if they were going to preface their prayer with the phrase, "If it be Thy will." Her relationship with God has always been deeply personal and sometimes feisty. I have been trying to learn after 27 years of marriage that I don't have to remake her in my image. In fact I realize I can learn a lot from her. She wrote of her take on this issue of God's will:

> "When I would share what I thought the Lord was leading me to pray, to claim a promise of Joe's healing, people kept saying to me, "God's will be done." That phrase was in The Lord's Prayer, so at first I thought I couldn't argue with it. One morning I was reading the entire prayer and the rest of

the verse struck me. "Thy will be done on earth as it is in heaven." I remember thinking sarcastically, "Is melanoma in heaven?" My literalism was causing some real questioning, again. Of course the answer is NO! Melanoma is not in heaven, disease is not in heaven. I could sense that same smile He gave me when I saw the verse, "Abide in Me and ask whatever you wish and it will be done for you." He whispered in my Spirit; ask Me to bring heaven to earth for you. I began praying, "Thy will be done on earth as it is in heaven." I do not want to write a theological book on prayer. I guess I do not care if anyone thinks I interpret the Bible right. I just sensed I had the ground to go boldly to the throne of grace and ask for melanoma to be removed. I did and He worked."

And His will was done.

Chapter Eighteen

~~~

Tipping Point

Psalm 40:2 - He brought me up out of the pit of destruction, out of the miry clay, And He set my feet upon a rock making my footsteps firm.

At this point in the battle, I was fighting hard but growing weaker and more fatigued, but Terri was ready to charge the next hill. She began to press the oncologist about a chemotherapy cocktail he had mentioned. Because of my deteriorating condition, he had soured on the idea, saying, "Any chemo right now will probably kill him." She and I agreed that I was going to die anyway, so I might as well try it. Let me pause and mention that not all patients think this way. Doctors rightly caution that chemo treatments can crater the quality of the last days of an individual's life. So I don't fault my doctor for attempting to discourage me, especially since Stage IV metastatic melanoma is not very responsive to chemo. Ultimately, I think the patient should make the decision without being pressured. I had always viewed chemo as avoidable and a last resort. Now from the human standpoint, I was pinning all my hopes on it. I figured I had nothing to lose. The doctor would later say that was the day Terri saved my life. He said I was too weak for outpatient chemo, so they kept me at the hospital for the four days of infusions. The chemo cocktail was developed at MD Anderson Cancer Center in Houston, TX, a highly regarded cancer center. The brew consisted of Taxol, a common breast cancer chemo; cistplatin, derived from the metal platinum; and dicarbazine (DTIC) which is used for many cancers. Taxol appealed to me because its tumor inhibitors were discovered from the bark of a rain forest tree, and natural elements were still utilized in its manufacture.

As soon as the Taxol hit my system, my doctor's warnings flashed through my mind. My breathing stopped and my heart seemed to skip several beats. I tried to sit up and attempted to speak, but could not. I tried to get out of the bed. I think I was trying to jump start my system which seemed to be shutting down. Terri and the nurses got very panicky, but grabbed me and made me lie down. They gave me massive doses of Benadryl and other drugs until my vitals settled. After that initial episode, the remainder of the first round went smoothly. My hair started to fall out in huge clumps but at least the nausea was minimal.

For some reason, the second round of chemo was much more intense than any of the other five rounds. As I rode home after the final treatment of round two, the serious vomiting began. Over that weekend in May 2003, I either vomited or had diarrhea (sometimes simultaneously) every ten to fifteen minutes for two full days. Just when I thought there was nothing left to purge, more would come forth. My epiglottis, the miniature "punching bag" structure which hangs down in the back of the throat, was so covered with gastric juices that it lost all rigidity. It sagged down and began restricting my air supply. Lower down my esophagus, the valve that separates the functions of breathing and eating was gummed up and not closing fully. As a result, my lungs began taking on acidic fluid from my stomach. I gasped for each breath between episodes of retching. My xiphoid process, the cartilage tab at the bottom of the sternum, became very irritated from the heaving. It is still damaged today and pops when I do a sit up. We frantically ordered prescriptions for every anti-nausea drug known to man, including Zofran and all the liquids and suppositories. I thought I might die of asphyxiation. I probably should have gone to the hospital, but I decided the car or ambulance ride might only worsen my condition. Nothing slowed down this purge, but ironically, this two day period marked the turning point.

I noticed the two walnut-sized masses under my skin by my collar bone had begun to shrink. By the end of the next week, they were totally gone. Naturally, we were elated and very encouraged. An oncologist wouldn't customarily prescribe a PET or CAT scan until after the final round of chemo, but Terri insisted and the doctor agreed to order a scan after round two of six. She was animated that the Lord was healing me and she wanted Him to get the glory, and not the chemo. I was convinced the Lord was miraculously healing me too … but through the chemo. The results came back; there was "significant shrinkage." Still, there was one huge warning in the report. Though the small mass on my pancreas had shrunk, the large pancreatic mass had continued to grow. It was three inches wide and six inches long. This report did not surprise me, since I still could not digest any food or drink because of the pancreatic pain whenever I tried. For some reason, the chemo was killing the melanoma everywhere but the most crucial site.

Another surgery to remove this pancreatic mass was out of the question. I was too weak, and the tumor was entwined with the pancreas. Conventional radiation, another common treatment option for most cancers, was never seriously considered. I was told early and often that conventional radiation did not work very well on melanoma. A normal dose of radiation is around 200 units which is safe for healthy tissue and fatal to many types of cancer cells. To kill melanoma, radiation levels must be almost 4 times greater at 700 radiation units. These levels from conventional radiation equipment can induce irreparable damage to healthy tissue surrounding a tumor. Thankfully, we remembered our melanoma treatment mentor had told us about a brand new high dose radiation machine, called a Novalis™. The Novalis™ can drastically reduce damage to healthy tissue because it is able to "shape" a beam of high dose radiation. The system uses a CAT scan to map the precise location of a tumor or tumors. It then targets the tumor's contours, enabling the radiation units to be dialed up enough to kill the melanoma. The machine's arm shoots the tumor from three sides, rotating from the top, then to the side, and finally shooting up from under the table. The concept made perfect sense, but would it work on tumors in the pancreas? At that time, there were only five Novalis™ machines in the world.

Lance Armstrong, the world champion cyclist and cancer survivor, had some treatment done at Richardson Regional Cancer Center. After his successful treatment there he asked the Center what they needed and they requested a Novalis™. He arranged to have one donated to Richardson Regional, which is just seven miles from our home. We made some initial inquiries about the process and a nurse tried to set up a screening with the radiation oncologist. The initial appointment kept getting bumped since most days I wasn't able to get around. The nurse kept calling and pursuing me though, even after he learned I had multiple sites, which we had thought rendered me less suitable for guided beam. I have no idea why he persisted. Maybe the Novalis™ business was slow at first. I'm going with - the Lord moved him. He eventually said, "Just show up whenever you can and we will fit you in." We were intrigued this radiation might be perfect for the stubborn pancreatic mass. Our oncologist told us we were nuts when we told him we were going to interrupt the chemo for the radiation. He asked why we would stop when we were getting such an extraordinary response. Obviously, there are huge risks to go against a doctor's advice, but he hadn't even heard of the treatment. We have noticed that doctors tend to stick close to "the standard of care" playbook, which insulates them from some of the second guessing and, let's just say it, from lawsuits. Yet someone has to try out these new technologies. The treatments were painless, with no side effects and each of the five treatments lasted just five minutes. The treatment unfolded so smoothly that I figured it was probably worthless. Yet in less than a few days after the end of treatment, I was certain it had killed the tumor. The pancreas pain reduced dramatically and then stopped. I was able to eat real food again! A post radiation CAT scan confirmed that the mass had indeed shrunk significantly. My oncologist was still a bit skeptical, but because of all of the shrinkage, he predicted I would probably be able to live nine more months. He later said, "I thought you were crazy to stop the chemo for the guided beam radiation, but now I send everybody over there (to receive the guided beam radiation)."

Despite the amazing physical progress, I faced another hurdle - self-absorption. I've had several other cancer patients tell me this too. They were all women though, so this is somewhat embarrassing.

Maybe guys just don't admit this type of struggle. Anyway, I understand now why self-focus took over. I needed to be in tune with my body to stay ahead of the cancer and pain. Even routine tasks had become painful. So when Terri hit a bump or a pothole which I thought she could have dodged, I would let her know about it. Since there was little meat on my bones, the PET scan table felt like a slab of concrete. I had to lie still for 35 minute sessions and then again for another 20 minutes. They warned me, if I moved, the pictures would be blurred and useless. Once during a scan I had become so uncomfortable, I could handle it no longer and shifted my body. The scan was discarded and I had to repeat it. Then there were the needles. Since my lymph nodes were removed from under my left arm, they had to stop sticking that arm for fear of swelling or infection. So they only stuck the veins in my right arm, which eventually began to rebel. The veins would appear ready, but collapse away from the needle, or the needle would bounce off the scar tissue. It became common for me to be stuck eight or ten times, by several different nurses, until one succeeded. Twice med students couldn't locate major arteries, once for a "central line" in my neck for the Interleukin-2, and once for a PICC line under my right arm for the chemo. In both instances when the student failed, the teacher thought the problem was a lack of force. I realized arteries have their own special set of nerves, which reminded me of the jolt of a spark plug on a lawnmower.

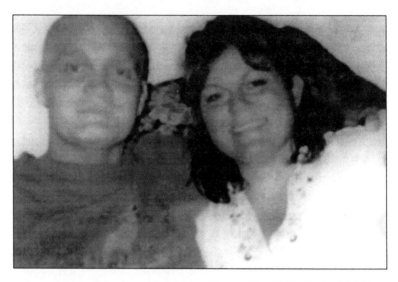

Joe during chemo with sister, Terry Gledhill (July 2003).

I mention all of this to explain why I felt so deserving of extra comfort. At first it felt good to let sadness reign and cry real good for myself. Let it out Joe, there, there, that's it, let it all out. I would rehash all the things I couldn't do. No preaching, basketball or fishing. For some reason I got particularly upset that I couldn't use the new barbecue grille which I had gotten on sale the previous fall. Soon I realized I had become addicted to self-pity, and it had become a dank and smelly dungeon. I longed to step outside of the cage. Self-pity is a foolish comfort, like bemoaning being in a ditch, while shoveling even more dirt out of the hole. "Look how deep I am now."

The Lord began to release me in an unexpected way. I asked my son, Jesse, to rent the entire DVD series, Band of Brothers, about Easy Company, the soldiers in the 101st Airborne during WWII. They had fought on D-Day from Normandy all the way into Germany. Watching their story was a wake up call for me. I wasn't freezing in a ditch in snowy woods on Christmas Eve, while being targeted all night by huge German artillery guns. I wasn't holding exploded buddies in my arms, trying to figure out what to say as they passed away. I wasn't left to waste away like an abandoned Jewish prisoner at Landsberg Concentration Camp. I had 100 times the support and 1000 times the comfort. The grit and sacrifice of those guys left me feeling foolish. Once I recalled asking my dad how he ended up in the army. I said, "So you were drafted, right?" No, he told me he signed up with the 101st Airborne on the day he graduated from high school. He and his buddies headed straight to the Army recruiting center as soon as school let out that summer. He would have joined sooner had he been allowed. Then there was me, Mr. Softy.

Another realization that shook me out of my self-pity was recognizing that some of the worst pain is emotional, not physical. I learned of someone who had experienced a very difficult betrayal. She strongly suspected her husband was having an affair. She confided in her best friend for months about her suspicion. Her best friend wondered aloud what she would do if it were true, and she wanted to know for a reason. You guessed it. Her best friend was the one having an affair with her husband. Emotional pain so intentionally and callously afflicted was much greater than what I was going through. My friend couldn't even talk about it for a couple of years as she attempted to salvage the marriage. With God's help, I decided to toughen up. Again I found the Lord to be my Stronghold. He pulled me up out of the miry clay of self-pity when I was hopelessly sinking down.

Chapter Nineteen

~~~

It's Gone!

Acts 3:7-8 - And seizing him by the right hand, he raised him up; and immediately his feet and his ankles were strengthened. With a leap he stood upright and began to walk; and he entered the temple with them, walking and leaping and praising God.

At the beginning of May 2003, my oncologist had told me I had just days to live. By early August, I was not merely surviving, I was rapidly recovering. I wondered if this was one of those brief remissions which we have all witnessed. Was the other shoe about to drop? My appetite returned and I found much of the 60 pounds I'd lost. My strength was increasing as well. On August 6th, I went fishing for a couple days with a good fishing buddy. Trust me; I applied a lot of sun screen. I was weak and couldn't cast very far. My grip was weak and once when I cast, my pole flew out of my hand into the water, but it didn't go very far. We laughed and fished the rod out of the water. I was getting my life back.

In mid-August after the third round of chemo, I had another PET scan. Afterwards, we took the films home because we were trying to keep my records together. Naturally, we snuck a peak at the films, but were shaken to see so many dark blotches on the pictures. I had "learned" that dark spots on the films signal an increased uptake of the radioisotope/glucose contrast. This is because fast growing cancer cells drink the contrast up at a greater rate than healthy cells. So it was evident to us the cancer had spread with a vengeance. The next day as I was receiving my fourth round of chemo, the doctor found Terri in the hall in a puddle of tears. She told him what we had seen on the scan, so he wanted to view them too. He came into my treatment room and hung the film on the backlight. He quickly clarified that some of the dark spots were not from cancer, but simply areas of increased blood flow. "That's your heart, Joe." Still, he identified several new areas of cancer. As we deciphered the films, his nurse walked in and announced the written results from the radiologist had just arrived. We figured we already knew what the report said, so we didn't really pay her much attention. She was thrown off by our pessimism and ongoing attempts to interpret the pictures ourselves. Finally, she raised her voice and said, "If you would all just listen, I will read the radiologist's results. It says, 'Correlation of this study with a previous outside PET scan in April demonstrates complete resolution of the previously described metastatic lesions involving multiple areas of the body. This is a NORMAL PET scan.'" In other words, they could find no cancer at all! Our embarrassment was short-lived as we broke into laughter and tears. All I could think of was the impossible odds of overcoming what so many people and medical professionals thought was a death sentence. Jesus' words came to me, "There is nothing too hard for God – only believe." The Lord is truly bigger than anything! I give all the glory to Him, no man healed me, it could only have been God!

Later as Terri and I were laughing at our lack of faith, we recalled the humorous account in the Book of Acts in chapter 12. Church leaders were deep in prayer for Peter's release from prison. James had already been put to death by Herod and so they understandably feared for Peter's life. There was a knock at the door and it was Peter himself. He had just been miraculously sprung from prison by an angel. A servant girl named Rhoda was so excited to hear Peter's voice that she neglected to unbolt the gate and let him in. When she reported Peter's presence to the spiritual giants back in the prayer meeting, they promptly questioned her sanity; "You are out of your mind" (Acts 12:15). Finally, she went back out to let Peter in and they were all amazed. It's a good thing the Lord is bigger than our faith. Fortunately, unshakeable faith is not a requirement for a miracle.

After our euphoria settled, I announced to the doctor that since the cancer was gone, I was going to quit the chemo. I was tired of throwing up. I had developed such an aversion to the chemo that more than once I threw up in the treatment room before the nurses even hung the IV bag. Even two years after my last treatment, I would still get queasy when I drove past the chemo hospital. In the battle of mind versus matter, matter had definitely won. The doctor thought it was a horrible idea to quit. He said, "Many doctors believe when a clean PET scan occurs to someone in your situation, there are still millions of microscopic cancer cells floating around in your body. The cells are spread out and too small to show up on the scan, but each round of chemo kills about half of those cells. So I wouldn't quit now." I did the math and realized he thought the cancer would never entirely go away. The chemo nurses had a similar perspective for my situation. They too had seen clean scans before. Terri mentioned to one nurse that the entire group of chemo nurses seemed a bit pessimistic. One particularly bold nurse responded, "We are not being pessimistic, just realistic. I have been doing this for 14 years and have never seen anyone get well who has had melanoma as bad as you." Several of the other nurses came into to help "manage our expectations." All I can say, with all due respect to the wonderful, amazing oncology nurses out there, experience can be overrated.

Only the Lord knows for sure whether I "needed" the last three rounds of chemo. I do believe He used the first two rounds to cure me. I had a tangible, overwhelming response. I could feel the lumps near my collar bone shrink and dissolve away. Was it all about the chemo and the radiation? Let me answer in this way: I have referred advanced melanoma patients to my oncologist. They have walked in and said to him, "Give me whatever you gave Joe." Later, during one of my follow-up appointments, my doctor said the chemo cocktail he gave me was not a wonder drug for Stage IV melanoma. He told me because of the amount of cancer, the size ("bulky"), and the locations of the spread of the disease, my "complete response" to the chemo was definitely a miracle. Some might conclude the chemo was just the right match for my particular strain and case of melanoma. "Sometimes the chemistry is just right and the medicine kicks in." I wonder if I had no treatment whatsoever, would the skeptic say, "Some people just get better and their cancer goes away for some unexplainable reason." I am content to adopt the conclusions of the medical people who work every day with dangerous cases of Stage IV melanoma. If they say this was a miracle, then that's my story!

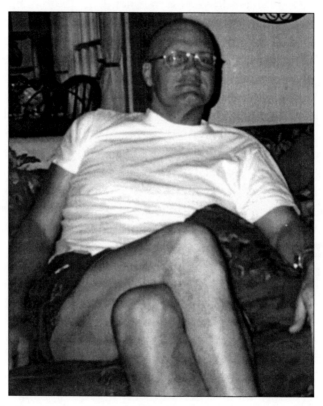

In September 2003, beginning to get back to normal after cancer is gone.

A couple in our church told me a story of an encounter they had with my surgeon who performed the three surgeries to remove my melanoma. I think their description of their meeting speaks volumes as to the supernatural nature of the healing:

In May of 2006, Mary *(not her real name)* was referred to a surgeon for varicose vein evaluation and treatment. On the Sunday before her first appointment, she mentioned to Joe's wife, Terri, that she was scheduled to see Dr. _____. Terri was excited, "He was Joe's surgeon! Be sure to tell him hello for us!"

After Mary was examined, she asked the doctor, "Do you remember Joe and Terri Fornear?"

The doctor replied, "Yes, of course I remember them. Why?"

"They said be sure to tell you hello for them."

"Are you telling me that Joe is still alive?"

"Sure, he is."

The doctor drew back, visibly paled, and totally astonished. "Why, when I saw him last, he was a dead man! For him to be alive is truly a miracle!"

The doctor became excited, opened the exam room door, and called his nurse in. "Remember Joe Fornear?" he asked.

"Yes, of course, I remember." She was equally stunned and elated by the news.

I was not convinced I needed the last three rounds of chemo, but just in case, I grunted them out. I finished the rounds during the next three months, until the end of October 2003. Then, just to be sure, I took some oral chemo pills called Temozolomide (Temador) and Thalidomide (Thalomid) until March of 2004. They had almost no side effects so I was very interested in them as adjuvants, which means they help keep the cancer from returning. Temador is often administered to brain cancer patients. It penetrates the brain/body barrier which not all chemos are effective in the brain. The Thalomid is famous, or infamous, for the birth defects it caused during the 1950's. It was used then for morning sickness, except it caused babies' limbs to grow partially, or not at all. Researchers later proved its value as a growth inhibitor on tumors. Even devastating tragedies can be turned to good use.

Part of the miracle of my healing was the speed at which I was recovering. On August 19th, I walked into the gym dressed for hoops.

My buddies were not sure what to do. They were glad to see me, but were clearly baffled that I might try to play. They kept saying, "Why are you dressed in your hoop clothes?" I was so skinny and bald and had that stylish, ashen gray glow from chemo. I had an IV line hanging out of my arm. So I cut off the foot portion of a white sock and used it as a sleeve to cover up and protect the line. I was there because I was trying to take my life back. After some bear hugs and handshakes, I tried to shoot the ball from about eight feet. The ball only went about four feet. I had to stand directly under the rim to finally make one. I was surprised by how much strength I had lost. This made me wonder if I should just hang out and not try to play, but when I saw they needed one more guy to make two full teams... I decided to be a good sport. I discovered quickly that my coordination needed some work. Twice that day, when I tried to backpedal down the court, I fell flat on my back. I had to remember to only run forward. The chemo line never got yanked out in the three months I was playing hoops and getting chemo treatments. The guys treated me with kid gloves for a while, but eventually they realized I had developed an annoying habit of stopping play so I could keep up. I would holler something like, "Time out, there is a wet spot on the floor down here." One day, one of the guys who has a speed game, said, "OK Joe, your cancer grace period is over. No more stopping play. If you need to take a break, you should get a substitute." I wasn't offended, he was right. This guy knew a thing or two about dealing with cancer. He had lost his wife to a fourteen year battle with breast cancer. So the grace period was officially over. Though I was feeling so much better, my appearance took some time to improve. At the kids "Meet the Teacher" event that August, several parents I knew passed me in the hall without greeting me. I knew we had made sufficient eye contact and I even said hello to several I thought I knew pretty well. When one parent introduced himself after talking with me for almost ten minutes, it hit me they didn't recognize me. My hair took some time to grow back, but trust me, my weight came back in a hurry. I had rediscovered food.

Chapter Twenty

~~~

Friends

Ecclesiastes 4:9-12 - Two are better than one because they have a good return for their labor. For if either of them falls, the one will lift up his companion. But woe to the one who falls when there is not another to lift him up. Furthermore, if two lie down together they keep warm, but how can one be warm alone? And if one can overpower him who is alone, two can resist him. A cord of three strands is not quickly torn apart.

Ask any cancer patient, one of the biggest pains about cancer is the i-word – insurance. You never really know what health insurance policy you have until you use it. I once read a quote that said, "Many plans are just like hospital gowns - you only think you're covered." Our health insurance strategy was a combination of policies. We had, and still have, a faith-based "need sharing" plan with Samaritan Ministries, out of Peoria, Illinois. This plan covered the first $100,000 of bills per incident, but it is not formally or legally called "insurance" and is not regulated by state insurance boards. Subscribers send their monthly "share" directly to other members who have incurred verifiable medical bills. Samaritan keeps medical costs low by subscribing regular churchgoers who don't use tobacco or illegal drugs and agree to practice "careful moderation" with alcohol. They must also sign an orthodox Christian statement of faith. On average, these restrictions drastically reduce individual's medical issues and costs. Under Samaritan's plan, my total out of pocket expense for the first $100,000 of cancer treatment was the initial "deductible" of $300! Every bill was paid and the subscribers prayed for me and sent me warm notes of encouragement. I have been with Samaritan now for 13 years. My family has had over 12 surgeries and I have never regretted using the Samaritan program. Downsides are the sheer number of checks that individuals send you to cover larger bills. The accounting can be a chore. Also, medical facilities usually consider Samaritan members to be "self-pay" and sometimes require money up front. But Samaritan works with you to front money to help pay bills until members checks arrive. Even with these drawbacks, I still highly recommend Samaritan.

Our plan to cover any bills over $100,000 was a Mutual of Omaha major medical plan with a $100,000 deductible. During the sales pitch with the Omaha agent, I missed the part about the deductible being "per calendar year" and not "per occurrence." I distinctly remember asking if the policy was seamless with the Samaritan program and at the time, even Samaritan was recommending this Omaha policy. The agent assured me there were no loopholes, fine print or surprises. I had several thousands of dollars of bills at the end of 2002 which used up a fair portion of Samaritan's $100,000 coverage. Then after I used up the balance of that $100,000 coverage early in 2003, there was a gap in coverage, because Omaha had reset my deductible back to $100,000 at the beginning of 2003. So I was responsible for the difference, thousand of dollars of bills before Omaha would begin coverage. The Omaha policy was useful in 2003 when I had the bulk of my treatment, with the costs easily exceeding the $100,000 deductible. But in 2004 and subsequent years, I would not have received a dime until bills in each of those calendar year exceeded $100,000. Then, the calendar year issue became a moot point when Omaha sent me a letter stating they would cancel my policy at the beginning of 2004. When I appealed to the State of Texas Insurance Board, they said Mutual was allowed to cancel the policy because they were cancelling the entire class of policies, not just mine. So everyone who had that policy was dropped. Well, that made me feel better. I never knew insurers could do that – a scary thought for us consumers.

Fortunately, most states, including Texas, have high risk insurance pools that cover this scenario. The premiums, co-pays and deductibles were very high though, averaging over $2000 a month for me alone. I mentioned this struggle to a brother and a friend and received an immediate and generous outpouring of help. My Pittsburgh family and an old friend from high school held a golf fundraiser in Pittsburgh. I was truly overwhelmed by the generosity of my family, high school friends from Upper St. Clair, and even my old Behrend College baseball teammates. Behrend is a branch campus of Penn State University in Erie, Pennsylvania. Then another friend from high school, held a benefit concert for me in Pittsburgh, which raised a very helpful chunk of money. My basketball buddies in Dallas held a generous fundraiser too; they called it "Free Throws for Joe."

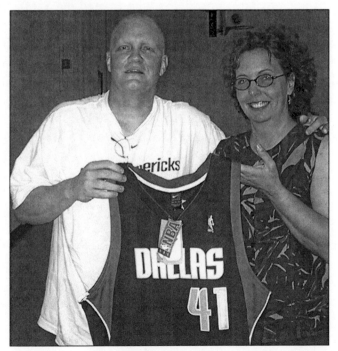

Joe and Terri after "Free Throws For Joe" fundraiser in November, 2003.

Then people from my church really kicked in to help too, and they graciously kept paychecks flowing throughout the whole ordeal. These funds covered all of my medical bills and insurance costs, plane trips, supplemental treatments and non-covered follow-up scans and treatments. Some folks mentioned to me later that they wanted to raise more money, but I told them no. They had helped me get back on my feet and I am forever grateful. You cannot imagine what a huge relief it was to Terri and me. We didn't have to worry about money, and we didn't plunge into debt, like so many of the medical horror stories I have heard. We were able to focus on getting the right treatment and not on cutting corners. I felt undeserving of such an outpouring, particularly with the Pittsburgh folks, because as I mentioned previously, I had not kept up with them very well. It was also humbling too, to accept so much generosity. I know I can never repay all those people.

About a year later, I noticed in the Samaritan Ministries guide-lines that they reinstate subscribers who exceed the $100,000 limit after a year of no evidence of a previously covered disease. So I called them and they reinstated me and agreed to cover cancer if I ever had a recurrence. I was already paying the top family rate with Samaritan so this renewed coverage didn't even cost any extra. My friends and family had gotten me over the hump. What a blessing! I could not miss the lesson here; sometimes the Lord's strong hold on us is through the extended hands of other people.

Chapter Twenty One

~~~

Purpose of It All

Luke 22:32 - I have prayed for you, that your faith may not fail; and you, when once you have turned again, strengthen your brothers.

People often tell me the Lord spared my life because He has a very special purpose for me. Many who observed my decline and recovery were totally amazed and their faith was definitely built up as a result. So I thought publishers, the medical world and the media would want to hear the story, and that my church would grow to 10,000 people. Yet that was not the plan the Lord had in mind. I don't wish to diminish the opportunities that I have had to share my story, because every invitation is an honor, but I was puzzled that people seemed to want to hear less, not more. One guy called to ask why I was sharing so many personal details in e-mails. A pastor cautioned me that his people often bored him with details of all their physical problems, so I should be careful. More than once my wife touched my leg under the table, or gave me "the glance," that my latest captive audience was fading fast. Recounting the details in a blow by blow fashion was therapeutic to me, especially right after the big turnaround. I was flipping emotional cartwheels everywhere I went. Yet I reluctantly concluded I was "over-sharing." I won't go as far as Mark Twain, who said, "Don't tell people your troubles; 95% of them don't care and the other 5% think you had it coming to you," but I have learned to scale back the tale considerably. Now I try to keep it short, saying, "I had melanoma in 14 different spots. The doctors gave me days to live and now the cancer is all gone. The Lord miraculously healed me." I provide further details when asked, but few people do. They get it pretty quickly and are glad for me. This is not a problem though, since the goal, after all, is that they be impressed by the Lord. Hopefully, hearing of a modern day miracle can inspire their faith in some way.

Though I struggled to discover what my healing meant with the general public, there was and is a wide open forum for my story. It is with cancer patients, particularly advanced melanoma patients. There is something about connecting with someone who has been through that grinder. Many cancer patients have a need to talk, to trade war stories, show scars and salve the emotional wounds. Surprisingly, I have found that I don't even have to be very profound; many are very encouraged that I am still breathing. I realized my ordeal was preparation for a new purpose and direction. I count it a privilege to be called to give back. After 18 years of pastoring, I decided to resign to start a non-profit ministry which we have named Stronghold Ministry. There is contact info at the back of this book. We counsel and encourage cancer patients, caretakers and their families. I see the difference that first-hand knowledge and empathy can bring to many patients. I have seen the peace of Almighty God fall on patients after I encourage them. I say, "It's understandable you feel depressed. You have been through so much with all the drugs and pain and treatments. You are seriously ill; no wonder you don't feel good. Don't worry; the Lord is your Stronghold. He is holding on to you right now and He won't let you go." I am honored that I have been called to be there for people. During my days of hand to hand combat, I wished I had someone to help unpack my doubts about faith, suffering and dying. Not all cancer patients are eager to talk though. Some are quite private and do not even open up with loved ones, let alone strangers. Many of these patients will never call or write, but we hope to try to reach them too through books and our website. We have a burden to assist caretakers as well. Their needs are often considered only as an afterthought in the midst of all of the turmoil.

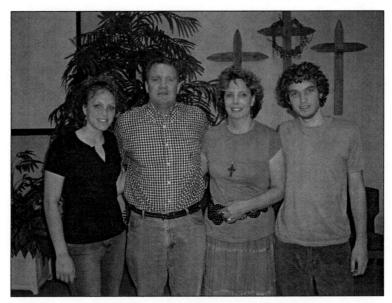

Joe and Terri with kids, Jesse and Amy.

There are many rewarding aspects of our ministry. We have had the sheer joy of laying hands on cancer patients and being part of their prayer support and have witnessed a few healings. I have also had opportunity to be a spiritual guide for cancer patients, steering them into the arms of the only Savior, Jesus Christ, just before they passed away. We have learned, however, that this ministry can exact an emotional toll, but that is a small price. I am inspired by the apostle, Paul, who said he would gladly go to hell for eternity in exchange for his fellow countrymen to go to heaven (Romans 9:3). If he would give up his eternal salvation, it is a small price for me to endure my own bout with cancer, and the emotional ups and downs of cancer ministry to help even one person end up in heaven for eternity. So, let me offer an invitation now. We would be delighted to make a connection with you or a loved one who needs support in their cancer or crisis. Please don't hesitate to connect with us. Our contact info is at the end of this book. And don't worry; I won't relate all my medical details to you - unless you ask!

Chapter Twenty Two

~~~

False Alarm(s)

Acts 9:16 - I will show him how much he must suffer for My name's sake.

After being miraculously healed from cancer, I assumed I'd suffered enough and paid my dues. I figured I had earned a medical exemption for the remainder of my days on the earth. But during a follow-up PET scan a year and a half later, radiologists saw some inflammation and a golf ball sized mass in a PET scan. This mass was in a suspicious location. It was in the middle of the surgical bed where they had removed a large cancerous lymph node and a third of my stomach that had the melanoma lesion. My oncologist told us there was a problem found on the scan. He sent me straight to a gastroenterologist to set up an endoscopy for pictures of the inside of my stomach. As we sat with the gastro doctor, he silently read the radiologist's report and looked up and told us the cancer had returned. Terri and I had driven separately to the appointment that day. On the way home, as we stopped at red lights, I would pull alongside her and catch her bawling. When she saw me watching, she would act strong, but I knew what she was thinking: "Here we go again, but will we dodge the bullet this time?" For a couple of days, we lived under that familiar black cloud. They decided to rescan me. The radiologist report mentioned my stomach may not have been sufficiently distended, or blown up. Evidently, before the first scan, I did not drink enough barium and my stomach had a little fold that mimicked a mass. The second scan was totally clean. They said stainless steel surgical clips probably caused the inflammation. The clips were used to permanently tie off veins after removing part of my stomach. I have seen the clips in CT scans, and no, they don't set off airport security scanners. So it was just a false alarm, but of course it was very troubling.

I have heard it said, "Once a cancer patient always a cancer patient." A doctor who had cancer wrote a book called something like, "Never Just a Headache Again." His theme was that after having cancer, every ache seems to signal the end of the remission. Most cancer patients can relate. In February of 2006, after I developed a persistent, banging headache, I thought I might have a brain tumor. My oncologist ordered an MRI of my brain. There was no smoking gun on the painful left side of my head, but there was a pea-sized mass above my right eye. He said I had a brain tumor and it should be immediately biopsied. He was preparing to find a surgeon to perform a long needle biopsy. He suggested my eye might need to be temporarily popped out to access the mass. I remembered having several sets of MRI films of my brain at home, so I suggested we compare the older films to see if this was a new object. He agreed, and we spent another day with that sinking feeling. The next day, after comparing with the older films and seeing no growth, the radiologist declared the mass benign. Another false alarm; it was probably "just a cyst".

Though I was cleared for cancer, I still had the banging headache. For four months, I went to specialists of all kinds, including a dentist, an ophthalmologist and an ENT doctor (ear, nose and throat). Eventually, it was determined I had "Eagle's Syndrome." A doctor named Eagle first diagnosed this rare disease in 1937. A ligament which is connected to the styloid bone at the base of the skull behind the ear, can calcify and press against veins and arteries or nerves. Mine was pressing against the jugular vein and a nerve which travels into my brain. The treatment called for surgery to clip the ligament from inside the mouth behind the tonsil area. Or the ligament can be clipped at the other end at the hyoid bone in the throat. The hyoid bone stacks on top of what we call "the Adam's apple." As I called around, it was evident that few doctors in Dallas had even heard of the syndrome, so it took some searching to find anyone who had actually performed the surgery. Finally I found a doctor who told me he had performed the procedure eight times with 100% success, so he was my man. The four inch incision he made on my neck was barely visible since it blended with the age line. No one knows for sure why this ligament hardens. This surgeon suggested the chemo and Interleukin-2 may have caused mine. After I recovered, I had relief from the headaches. So once again, I encouraged the Lord to grant me a long break from medical issues and pain.

The prayer for relief was not yet answered. In the beginning of 2008, a pain in my abdomen grew more intense by the day. I finally told Terri and my oncologist. We all wondered if the cancer had come back, but I was convinced it was my stomach surgery staples. I had a total work up and they found no smoking gun. So now I figured everyone would think I just had a dramatic flair. I couldn't blame them. I wondered myself at times. Twice I stopped taking the pain pills just to see what would happen, but the pain was real. Eventually, I was taking 10 hydrocodones a day, and I still had pain. Something had to give, so I began pressing a surgical oncologist to perform exploratory surgery. He told me he was suspicious the cancer had returned and insisted on new scans. I had just been scanned, but I decided to get the scans to comply with his process. When the new scans came back clean, he was still reluctant to do the exploratory surgery. When I told him the pain increased with sitting, he suggested I try a lifestyle change, like standing up all day. So I found another surgeon who was willing to perform laparoscopic exploratory surgery. A friend who was in med school at the time recommended a bariatric surgeon who was known for successfully tackling stomach surgery complications. This doctor thought I probably had an "adhesion" from my previous stomach surgery. Adhesions are common after surgery because tissue and organs become sticky and adhere to one another. He said there was a 50-50 probability that unsticking my insides would cure the pain. While researching adhesions, I found a private foundation in England which was devoted to educating the medical community about adhesions. They said many people with persistent adhesions, especially women, are commonly sent to the psych ward. When scans show no problems, many doctors conclude there must be some psychosomatic elements at work. Honestly, by the way that first surgical oncologist looked at me, I could tell he wondered if I had some issues.

So in February 2008, the bariatric doctor pumped up my abdomen with air, and with the aid of a tiny camera, cut loose all the adhesions from the wall of my abdomen. He said my omentum was sticking to the inside of my abdominal wall and pinching some nerves. The omentum is a body part made popular by Oprah's doctor – Dr. Oz. It is the fat layer which cushions and insulates our internal organs. After the surgery, my pain stopped in a week. At one of the lower points of this medical trial, I pleaded with the Lord for an extended season of no pain. Why did He heal me of cancer, only to face these chronic false alarms, complications and more pain? In James 1:5-8, He promises wisdom in the midst of our trials:

> But if any of you lacks wisdom, let him ask of God, who gives to all generously and without reproach, and it will be given to him. But he must ask in faith without any doubting, for the one who doubts is like the surf of the sea, driven and tossed by the wind. For that man ought not to expect that he will receive anything from the Lord, being a double-minded man, unstable in all his ways.

I believe the Lord answered my cry for wisdom by illuminating a Bible passage. In Acts 9, Jesus had tired of Saul's (renamed Paul) persecution of His new church. He wanted Saul to work for Him, not against Him. So while en route to imprison more Christians, Jesus knocked him off his horse. To help guide Saul into his new life's work, the Lord spoke to a man named Ananias. Jesus said about Paul, "He is a chosen instrument of Mine, to bear My name before the Gentiles and kings and the sons of Israel; for I will show him how much he must suffer for My name's sake" (Acts 9:15-16). I'm guessing Paul liked the first part of his calling much better than the second. To be God's chosen messenger to royalty and the masses would be an honor, but why was suffering so necessary to carry Christ's name? Could God use Paul without all the suffering? I believe the Lord spoke to me through this verse. He had been allowing ongoing suffering so I might tell of His power in the cancer and medical communities. He knew they weren't likely to come to me, so He was sending me back to them. I showed up, not as some amazing case study at a medical conference, but as a hurting patient. Since patient history is always part of the work-up drill, I have had numerous opportunities to share my story, well, His story. I have shared the Lord in depth with some doctors and medical staff. To some I have given them my gospel tract, "The Two Ways to Get to Heaven" (see Appendix). Mostly, I have been able to tell them about the Lord healing me from multiple site, Stage IV metastatic melanoma. Most agree it was a miracle. They know metastatic melanoma is an aggressive cancer. But also, God knows the cancer and general medical community need encouragement. They are God's hands on the earth. They constantly treat patients with long treatment odds. I'm sure their prayers for patients are countless. They need to know that sometimes He answers their prayers in amazing ways.

God knows, I want my life to be smooth sailing. Not smooth by and by and in the end, but by the end of today! Most people share this desire, but the wish will always be fantasy. Acts 14:22 deals with this notion with such bluntness, it is almost humorous. After founding many churches across Greece and eastern Asia, Paul and his fellow leaders decided to revisit and strengthen these churches. What encouraging word would you have delivered? How about this message: "Through many tribulations we must enter the kingdom of God"? Now there's a pick-me-up for you. I suppose grasping the fact that hardship is part of life is, as they say, half the battle. Paul's trials were numerous, but he had such a liberating attitude about life's troubles. In 2 Corinthians 11:24-27, he describes some of the trials he endured:

> Five times I received from the Jews thirty-nine lashes. Three times I was beaten with rods, once I was stoned, three times I was shipwrecked, a night and a day I have spent in the deep. I have been on frequent journeys, in dangers from rivers, dangers from robbers, dangers from my countrymen,

dangers from the Gentiles, dangers in the city, dangers in the wilderness, dangers on the sea, dangers among false brethren; I have been in labor and hardship, through many sleepless nights, in hunger and thirst, often without food, in cold and exposure.

Paul was in trouble with authorities so frequently that even his loyal followers began to doubt his credibility. In the book of 2 Timothy 1:16, Paul complimented a man named Onesiphorus because, "He often refreshed me and was not ashamed of my chains." Obviously, some of his followers were ashamed of his chains. I imagine some people thought Paul might be a pretty decent leader if he weren't in jail all the time. I also wondered if Paul ever sheepishly asked the Lord the obvious question, "Haven't I suffered enough?" He tells us he prayed three times for God to remove these trials from his life. I take it he meant he engaged in three "seasons" of prayer, not just three separate prayers. Don't ask me how long a season is: it's just longer than a single prayer. He called these trials his "thorn in the flesh," and as far as we know, the constant irritations never subsided until the day he too was crucified on a cross. God answered Paul, saying, "My strength is perfected in weakness." Later, Paul made peace with his troubles. He declared in 2 Corinthians 12:10, "Therefore, I am well content with weaknesses, with insults, with distresses, with persecutions, with difficulties, for Christ's sake; for when I am weak, then I am strong." This attitude is not just for super Christians and full time ministers; he is describing what should be the "normal" Christian attitude. Who can muster up that type of endurance and strength? The answer is no one can. You see, the Christian life was never intended to be lived by anyone other than Jesus Christ Himself. This is why Paul says in Galatians 2:20 that it is actually Christ who lives the Christian life <u>through</u> him.

I have been crucified with Christ; and it is no longer I who live, but Christ lives in me; and the life which I now live in the flesh I live by faith in the Son of God.

So the secret to handling great trials is letting Christ's life within us do the coping. This lesson sometimes eludes me, but the Lord keeps giving new opportunities to learn. In fact, as I was finalizing this book, two new medical issues arose. (I need to hurry up and get this book completed). First, I blew out two discs in my back playing basketball. Then the Eagle's Syndrome returned with a vengeance. I had another surgery, this time to break off the styloid bone which had grown over one inch too long and was rubbing on my jugular and a brain nerve. So I am still taking laps in the wilderness, but at least I can make sense of why it is happening. My curriculum in the school of suffering has been designed for me to master weakness, or rather to master my "strength". I can't say I like feeling weak. It feels so un-American and weakness runs counter to my roots in the Steel City of Pittsburgh. I want to be strong and capable and demonstrate "the triumph of the human spirit," but God is more concerned about showing His power than mine.

I recall when I was in college, a Christian leader whom I really admired, had a very painful experience when his appendix burst. He described the ordeal and explained how much it drew him to the Lord. I began hoping God would give me a bout with appendicitis too. When I shared my wish with this leader, he said, "Oh Joe, I wouldn't wish that on anyone. God knows how to draw you to Himself. He will give you your own experience." Indeed He has, but I would have settled for a busted appendix. But God always knows what He is doing. He has prepared me to help others as He has helped me.

Blessed be the God and Father of our Lord Jesus Christ, the Father of mercies and God of all comfort, who comforts us in all our affliction so that we will be able to comfort those who are in any affliction with the comfort with which we ourselves are comforted by God. For just as the sufferings of Christ are ours in abundance, so also our comfort is abundant through Christ. But if we are afflicted, it is for your comfort and salvation; or if we are comforted, it is for your comfort, which is effective in the patient enduring of the same sufferings which we also suffer; and our hope for you is firmly grounded, knowing that as you are sharers of our sufferings, so also you are sharers of our comfort.

If you ever want someone to comfort you and encourage you in the midst of serious illness, look me up. By now, you know my core message: When it seems like you're losing your grip, remember He has got a stronghold on you. Oftentimes, talking out your struggles can bring great comfort. Don't let my struggles go to waste.

Chapter Twenty Three

~~~

Back to "Normal"

Psalm 90:10 - As for the days of our life, they contain seventy years, Or if due to strength, eighty years, Yet their pride is but labor and sorrow; For soon it is gone and we fly away.

In most areas, my life is back to normal. Small talk has returned. For a time, when someone asked how I was doing, we both knew it was a question about my survival chances. Yet the medical people say, if a Stage IV metastatic melanoma patient survives for five years with No Evidence of Disease (NED), they are out of the woods. On August 13, 2008, I reached that five year milestone. So if melanoma rears its ugly head again, it will be a new case and not a recurrence. I am still amazed that I am alive. In my ministry to cancer patients, I have observed how devastating cancer can be. I am extremely grateful to the Lord first, and grateful for all of the practical help and support of my friends and family. What a blessing!

People sometimes ask if I approach life differently now. Though I am far from macrobiotic, I have definitely changed in a few very practical ways. I eat better and less. I work fewer hours. I lather on sun screen thicker, and repeat more. By no means did the healing catapult me to a higher level of spirituality. Is it really easy now to stay on track? The short answer is no. Each day, I have to try to grab my drift-prone soul to focus on what is most important. My near death experience forced me to face life's vanities and empty pursuits.

In those days when I lay dying, I really "saw" my own shallow-ness. How I was too concerned with achievements and status. I also caught a glimpse of what total relief will be like. Frankly, I have to be careful with that vision when life is hard. There was a time during the battle when I totally let go of this life and "tried on" heaven. But just as I began to be enthralled by the comfort of that silky garment, I was told to take it off. I seek to keep that vision of heaven fresh, but without clinging to it. I want my remaining days to impact others for the Lord and His eternal purposes. I've been to the edge of life and death and I was overwhelmed by the sheer brevity of this life. Like a blade of desert grass which pops up in the cool morning and withers under the piercing heat of the sun, our days fly by so quickly. Moses prayed in Psalm 90:12, "Teach us to number our days, that we may present to You a heart of wisdom." It is normal to die. We all live with that fact, but the wise live in preparation for that day. I'm trying to live this moment for that moment. Most of us know and believe there are extra rewards offered in heaven for more faithful living here on earth. So living for the next life only makes sense. Are you ready to die? No matter what path you have chosen thus far in your life, do yourself a favor, get into, and stay in His grip. Let's not waste another day!

Appendix One

~~~

The Two Ways to Get to Heaven

Are You Heaven Bound?

90% of Americans believe in heaven— and a whopping 85% believe they will go to heaven when they die according to an ABC news poll on October 5, 2005). Yet how do we know for sure if we will go to heaven? This should not be a guessing matter. After all, heaven and hell last for eternity.

God Himself wants us to know *now* how to get to heaven. That is why He left us a written, objective record of His thoughts so we would not be in the dark. This record is the Bible—His Word. The apostle John stated the purpose for which he wrote, "I write to you so that you may know that you have eternal life" (I John 5:13). So, consider now the two ways to get to heaven.

Plan A: Be perfect

If you want to be judged based on your deeds, Galatians 3:10 clearly sets out the requirements: "For as many as are of the works of the Law are under a curse; for it is written, 'Cursed is everyone who does not abide by all things written in the book of the law to perform them.'" So to avoid the curse of the law, which is eternal hell, and go to heaven, you must have never, ever failed to obey all the things written in the Law. Honestly now, have you ever lied, cheated on a test, stolen from someone or a store, cursed, lusted in your heart, been unkind or unforgiving, gossiped, gotten drunk or had sex outside of marriage? If you have ever sinned in any of these ways, forget about Plan A—it's already too late.

The Bible says: "For whoever keeps the whole law and yet stumbles in <u>one</u> point, he has become guilty of all" (James 2:10). Think about this simple illustration that may help you understand falling short of heaven by failing to obey. Some of us may be able to leap across a narrow ravine, but to get to heaven by our deeds none of us can leap across the Grand Canyon of total perfection. We all fall short. "All have sinned and fallen short of the glory of God" (Romans 3:23).

So are you ready for "Plan B"?

Plan B: Believe

Fortunately God has made a way for us to go to heaven apart from our performance. It is the way of faith—believing in Jesus Christ alone. As God says in Romans 4:5, "To the one who does not work, but believes in Him (Jesus) who justifies the ungodly, his faith is credited as righteousness."

So why does God present Jesus Christ as the object of faith? Romans 5:8-9 explains, "God demonstrates His own love toward us, in that while we were yet sinners, Christ died for us. Much more then, having now been justified by His blood, we shall be saved from the wrath of God through Him." It is simple, Christ died in our place so we might be forgiven.

Romans 6:23 captures our options well: "For the wages of sin is death, but the free gift of God is eternal life in Christ Jesus our Lord." Did you notice that eternal life (going to heaven) is called a "free gift"? Is there a catch? No, Jesus Himself said in John 3:16, "For God so loved the world, that He gave His only begotten Son, that whoever believes in Him shall not perish (or go to hell), but have eternal life (go to heaven)."

So how do you receive this free gift?

Receive

The Bible has some very good news regarding how to receive this free gift of eternal life. In John 1:12 we read, "But as many as received Him, to them He gave the right to become children of God, even to those who believe in His name." Receiving Christ is believing in Him as God's only Savior from your sin. He took upon Himself the penalty of your sin, which is death—that is why He had to die on the cross. But you have to personally receive His work on the cross to have your sins forgiven and allow your entry into heaven. So talk to God. Admit you are not good enough, that you have sinned against Him. Then receive His solution to your sin problem. Do yourself a huge favor and don't delay this decision to receive Jesus Christ even one minute!

After you receive Christ, turn your whole life over to Him. He said that He came to give abundant life—a full and satisfying life so you can trust Him with everything. Then get committed to a good Bible teaching church so that you can grow in your new faith.

If you have received Christ after reading this tract, please let me know, I want to encourage you and send you some free information on following Jesus Christ.

Appendix Two

~~~

Information on Melanoma

Disclaimer: Please understand the following information is not professional medical advice. Please verify all information with your doctor.

Little known facts about melanoma:

- Babies have been born with melanoma.
- Melanoma lesions can appear on the skin, spread cancerous cells to nearby lymph nodes (Stage III) and then disappear quickly from the skin. (This happened to me, Joe Fornear).
- Melanoma lesions don't have to be big to be dangerous. (Joe's father, Bob, had an advanced case of Stage IV and had only a very small "primary" or original source lesion on his back).
- Melanoma can first appear on or in a person's eye.
- Ultraviolet rays from the sun can penetrate light clothing, and melanoma lesions have been found in areas where bathing suits cover the skin, especially true for women. Some women have been diagnosed with melanoma on their private area.
- In men, melanoma most often shows up on the upper body, between the shoulders and hips and on the head and neck.
- In women, melanoma often develops on the lower legs.

- In dark-skinned people, melanoma often appears under the fingernails or toenails, on the palms of the hands or on the soles of the feet.

Melanoma - Most Common Signs and Symptoms:

Melanoma is the most dangerous form of skin cancer, caused by a malignancy of the melanocytes, the cells that produce pigment in the skin. Melanoma is most common in people with fair skin, but can occur in people with any skin color. Most melanomas present as a dark, mole-like spot that spreads and, unlike a mole, has an irregular border. The tendency to contract melanoma is considered to be inherited by some oncologists, but the risk increases with over-exposure to the sun and sunburn.

One of the most important variables in successfully treating melanoma is early diagnosis. Often the first sign of melanoma is a change in the size, shape, color, or feel of an existing mole. Most melanomas have a black or blue-black area. Melanoma also may appear as a new mole. If you have a question or concern about something on your skin, immediately see a skin doctor, called a dermatologist, or a cancer doctor, called an oncologist.

The acronym, "ABCD" is a good tool to help you remember what to watch for:

- * Asymmetry— The shape of one half of a mole does not match the other.
- * Border— The edges are often ragged, notched, blurred, or irregular in outline; the pigment may spread into the surrounding skin.
- * Color— The color is uneven. Shades of black, brown, and tan may be present. Areas of white, grey, red, pink, or blue also may be seen.
- * Diameter— There is a change in size, usually an increase. Melanomas are usually, but not always, larger than the eraser of a pencil (1/4 inch or 5 millimeters).

<u>Staging and Treatment of Melanoma</u>: Staging is the process of determining the progress of the melanoma. To stage a patient, dermatologists and oncologists usually focus on three variables:

1. The thickness or depth of the tumor
2. Whether the tumor is ulcerated (cracked or bleeding)
3. If, and how far, the cancer cells have spread

<u>Stage I</u>

The lesion is thin and confined to the surface of the skin. It has not spread to any lymph nodes or other organs.

Treatment

The tumor and some surrounding tissue are removed surgically. Usually no further treatment is necessary.

<u>Stage II</u>

The lesion has spread to deeper layers of the skin. It has not spread to any lymph nodes or other organs.

Treatment

The tumor and some surrounding tissue, called a margin, are removed surgically. Sometimes an immunotherapy drug such as interferon is given in the case of thicker or larger lesions.

<u>Stage III</u>

The skin lesion may be any thickness, but cancer cells have spread to lymph nodes or other new areas on the skin near the original site.

Treatment

The tumor and some surrounding tissue, called a margin, are removed surgically. Also lymph nodes which have been affected are removed surgically. Immunotherapy drugs such as interferon or interleukin are given.

Stage IV

The cancer cells have spread past lymph nodes to other organs in the body, or areas far from the original site of the tumor. This is called metastatic melanoma.

Treatment

The skin lesion and cancerous lymph nodes are removed surgically. Radiation therapy, chemotherapy, or immunotherapy drugs such as interferon or interleukin are given. Often biochemotherapies are given, which is a combination of chemo and immunotherapies.

Appendix Three

~~~

Glossary – Medical Definitions

Adjuvant: Adjuvant therapy for cancer usually follows surgery to remove tumors or lymph nodes. Adjuvants are treatments, such as chemotherapy, immunotherapy or radiation, which are used to decrease the risk of recurrence, or return, of the cancer.

CT or CAT scan: Computerized tomography scan. Pictures of structures within the body are created by a computer that consolidates data from multiple X-ray images and converts them into pictures on a screen. The CT scan can reveal some soft-tissue and other structures that cannot be seen in conventional X-rays. A tomogram ("cut") is a picture of a slice of the body which can be made visible with 100 times more clarity than an X-ray.

Endoscopy: A lighted, flexible instrument which may also have a device for removing tissue for testing. The most common endoscopic procedures evaluate the throat, stomach, and portions of the intestine (colonoscopy).

Interferon: A naturally occurring bodily substance that "interferes" with the ability of viruses to reproduce. Can be synthetically reproduced for cancer treatment. Interferon boosts the immune system.

Interleukin-2: IL-2. A naturally occurring chemical messenger that can improve the body's response to disease. It stimulates the growth of certain disease-fighting cells in the immune system. It can be manufactured in the laboratory and used for cancer treatment.

MRI: Magnetic resonance imaging. Designed to image internal structures of the body using magnets, radio waves, and a computer to produce images of body structures. The scanner is a tube surrounded by a large circular magnet. The patient is placed on a moveable bed that is inserted into the magnetic field. A computer processes the information generated by radio waves which are bounced off the magnetized cells in the body, and an image is produced. The image and resolution is quite detailed and can detect tiny changes of structures within the body, particularly in the soft tissue, brain and spinal cord, abdomen and joints.

PET scan: Positron emission tomography. A specialized imaging technique that adds a short-lived radioactive tracer to intravenously injected glucose to produce three-dimensional colored images of the insides of the body. PET scanning provides information about the body's chemistry not available through other procedures. Unlike CT (computerized tomography) or MRI (magnetic resonance imaging), techniques that look at anatomy or body form, the PET studies metabolic activity or body function. The extent and location of cancer growth is measured because fast growing cancer masses soak up an injected mixture of glucose and a radioactive tracer at a greater rate than healthy tissue.

Appendix Four

~~~

Information on Stronghold Ministry

Stronghold Ministry was founded by Joe and Terri Fornear to provide spiritual support and comfort to cancer patients, caretakers and others in major life crisis. We reach out through personal contact, through the internet and via telephone. *Please don't hesitate to call us or to refer someone who wants some spiritual help!*

SERVICES

We provide counseling, host support groups, speak in home groups, Sunday school classes, youth groups and Joe can be a Sunday morning guest speaker at your church service. We host retreats and conferences as well.

COSTS

We offer our services free to cancer patients and those in crisis. Stronghold Ministry operates solely on donations. We have incorporated as a non-profit in the State of Texas and we have been granted a 501(c) 3 tax exemption by the IRS, so donations are tax deductible.

Contact Information

Website - www.mystronghold.org
E-mail – jfor@mystronghold.org
Phone: 214-641-8916

Joe also has a blog at: http://www.mystronghold.org/Blog/
Mailing address:
Stronghold Ministry
P.O. Box 38478
Dallas, TX 75238